The Pocket Doctor
2001

D1249107

The Pocket Doctor
2001

Michael S. Sherman, M.D.
Edward S. Schulman, M.D.
MCP Hahnemann School of Medicine

EDUCATIONAL COMMUNICATIONS
Mount Kisco, New York

The Pocket Doctor is intended as a quick and convenient reminder of information you have learned previously. Treatment recommendations are based on published clinical practice guidelines, reliable medical literature, and interpretation by our authors who are knowledgeable in their fields. Tables and algorithms are designed as a guide for uncomplicated patients and are not meant to substitute for sound clinical judgment and individualization of therapy. Though extensive efforts were made to assure accuracy and completeness, unerring treatment recommendations cannot be guaranteed. Moreover, *The Pocket Doctor* may contain typographical errors, omissions, and in certain instances, controversial treatment preferences of the authors.

In general, drug indications and dosages listed in *The Pocket Doctor* have been recommended in the medical literature and conform to the practices of the general medical community, rather than those of any specific institution, geographic region, or practice specialty. However, this does not imply approval of the United States Food and Drug Administration (FDA) for their use in the diseases and dosages listed. Package inserts for each drug should be consulted for the uses and dosages that are FDA approved. Also, because of constant modifications of indications and dosages, particularly of new drugs, it is necessary for the health care professional to keep abreast of such revised recommendations.

ISBN: 0-9672263-1-7

PRINTED IN THE UNITED STATES OF AMERICA

About our web site: www.PocketDoctor.com

In recognition of the rapidity of changes in medical knowledge, we have established a free internet site, **www.PocketDoctor.com.** This web site offers some of the individual algorithms that appear in the book version along with annotations on critical decision points and, where available, links to relevant source material. As we receive new information, guideline changes, and feedback from our readers, the editors and authors will modify individual algorithms and tables "on-line." Updates will be posted as changes are made. Please check this site regularly for updates. Registered users will be informed by e-mail when new material is added to the site. We plan to add a bulletin board in the near future. We welcome your comments and suggestions, which can be e-mailed through the site.

Contents

Contributors

Neil Aronin MD
Professor of Medicine and Cell Biology
University of Massachussetts Medical
Center

Ausim Azizi
Associate Professor of Neurology
MCP Hahnemann School of Medicine

Jack Becker MD
Assistant Professor of Pediatrics
Temple University School of Medicine

Thompson K. Boyd III MD
Assistant Professor of Medicine
Chairman, Utilization Review
MCP Hahnemann School of Medicine

Stephen Bulova MD
Staff Physician, Christiana Care Hopitals
Delaware Clinical and Laboratory
Physicians
Newark, Delaware

Harris Clearfield MD
Professor of Medicine
Division of Gastroenterology
MCP Hahnemann School of Medicine

James Conroy DO, FACP, FACOI
Professor of Medicine (ret)
Division of Hematology/Oncology
MCP Hahnemann School of Medicine

Jane Doszpoly MA, RD, CNSD
Department of Nutrition Services
Hahnemann University Hospital

Mary Elmer RN, CCRN, CRNP
Jefferson Medical College

Sol Epstein MD
Chief Medical Director
Roche Laboratories
Adjunct Professor of Medicine
University of Pennsylvania

Babak Etemad MD
Assistant Professor of Medicine
Medical University of South Carolina

Pierre B. Fayad MD
Associate Professor of Neurology
Yale University

Amy Chernoff Fuchs
Assistant Professor of Medicine
Division of Infectious Diseases
MCP Hahnemann School of Medicine

Barry Fuchs MD
Assistant Professor of Medicine
University of Pennsylvania School of
Medicine

Jeffrey Glassroth MD
George R and Elaine Love Professor and
Chair
Department of Medicine
University of Wisconsin Medical School

Jonathan E. Gottlieb MD
Associate Professor of Medicine
Division of Pulmonary and Critical Care
Jefferson Medical College
Senior VP, Clinical Affairs
Thomas Jefferson University Hospital

Scott Hessen MD
Assistant Professor of Medicine
Division of Cardiology
MCP Hahnemann School of Medicine

Susan Hoch MD
Associate Professor of Medicine
Lupus and Arthritis Center
MCP Hahnemann School of Medicine

David M. Hoenig MD
Assistant Professor of Urology
Montefiore Medical Center
Albert Einstein College of Medicine

Steven L. Hubert MD
Assistant Professor of Dermatology
MCP Hahnemann School of Medicine

Mercedes P. Jacobson MD
Director, Epilepsy Center
MCP Hahnemann School of Medicine

Draga Jichici HBSc, MD, FRCPC
Norfolk Medical Center
Guelf, Ontario

Margaret Khouri MD
Associate Professor of Medicine
Division of Gastroenterology
Texas Tech University Health Science
Center at Odessa

Robert Kotloff MD
Associate Professor of Medicine
Pulmonary, Allergy and Critical Care
Division
University of Pennsylvania School of
Medicine

Thomas Kowalski MD
Associate Professor of Medicine
Jefferson Medical College

David Kountz, MD
Associate Professor of Medicine
Chief, Division of Primary Care
UMDNJ-Robert Wood Johnson Medical
School

Donald Kushon MD
Assistant Professor of Psychiatry
MCP Hahnemann School of Medicine

Steven Kutalek MD
Associate Professor of Medicine
Chief, Division of Cardiology
MCP Hahnemann School of Medicine

David Lang MD
Associate Professor of Medicine
Director, Division of Allergy and Immunology
Jefferson Medical College

Alyssa A. LeBel MD
Assistant Professsor of Anaesthesiology
and Neurology
University of Pennsylvania School of
Medicine
Children's Hospital of Philadelphia

David C. Lee, MD, FAAEM
Clinical Assistant Professor
Department of Emergency Medicine
NYU School of Medicine
North Shore University Hospital

Frank Leone MD
Assistant Professor of Medicine
Director, Medical Respiratory Intensive
Care Unit
Thomas Jefferson University Hospital

Carlos M. Martinez MD
Assistant Professor of Medicine
Department of Family Practice
Bella Vista Hospital, Mayagüez, Puerto Rico

A. Scott Mathis, Pharm. D.
Clinical Assistant Professor
Rutgers College of Pharmacy
Rutgers University

Joseph McClellen MD
Director, Hamot Heart Institute
Erie, Pennsylvania

Geno Merli MD, FACP
Ludwig A. Kind Professor and
Acting Chair, Department of Medicine
Jefferson Medical College

John Morgan MD
Associate Director
Cardiovascular Disease Prevention Center
Jefferson Medical College

Thomas J. Nasca MD, FACP
Professor of Medicine and Dean
Jefferson Medical College

David Naide MD
Associate Professor of Medicine
Head, Section of Vascular Medicine
Division of Cardiology
MCP Hahnemann School of Medicine

Michael Niederman MD
Professor of Medicine
SUNY at Stony Brook
Chief, Pulmonary and Critical Care Division
Winthrop University Hospital

Olusola Osundeko MD
Fellow, Division of Endocrinology
MCP Hahnemann School of Medicine

Harold I. Palevsky MD
Professor of Medicine
University of Pennsylvania Medical Centers

Herbert Patrick MD
Associate Professor of Medicine
Director of Critical Care Services
MCP Hahnemann School of Medicine

Donald G. Raible MD
Clinical Associate Professor of Medicine
Division of Pulmonary and Critical Care
MCP Hahnemann School of Medicine

James Reynolds MD
Professor of Medicine and Chief,
Division of Gastroenterology and Hepatology
MCP Hahnemann School of Medicine

Leslie Rose MD
Professor of Medicine
Division of Endocrinology and Metabolism
MCP Hahnemann School of Medicine

Daniel Rukstalis MD
Associate Professor of Surgery and
Pathology
Urology Division
MCP Hahnemann School of Medicine

Jamie Ellen Siegel MD
Associate Professor of Medicine
Hematology Division
UMDNJ-Robert Wood Johnson Medical
School

Edward S. Schulman M.D.
Professor of Medicine and
Chief of Service
Pulmonary and Critical Care Medicine
Hahnemann University Hospital
MCP Hahnemann School of Medicine

Allan B. Schwartz MD
Professor of Medicine
Division of Nephrology
MCP Hahnemann School of Medicine

Kumar Sharma MD
Assistant Professor of Medicine
Division of Nephrology
Jefferson Medical College

Michael S. Sherman M.D.
Associate Professor of Medicine
Division of Pulmonary and Critical Care
MCP Hahnemann School of Medicine

Richard L. Spielvogel MD
Professor and Chair,
Department of Dermatology
MCP Hahnemann School of Medicine

Michael Styler MD
Associate Professor of Medicine
Division of Hematology/Oncology
MCP Hahnemann School of Medicine

Carole E. Thomas MD
Assistant Professor of Neurology
Director, Acute Stroke and Neurointensive
Care Program
MCP Hahnemann School of Medicine

Allan R. Tunkel MD, PhD
Professor of Medicine
MCP Hahnemann School of Medicine

James Witek M.D.
Assistant Professor of Medicine
Section of HIV/AIDS Medicine
MCP Hahnemann School of Medicine

Eric T. Wittbrodt, Pharm. D.
Assistant Professor of Clinical Pharmacology
Philadelphia College of Pharmacy
University of the Sciences in Philadelphia

Preface

"Memory is treacherous. It is particularly so with those who have much to do and more to think of. When the best remedy is wanted . . . it is difficult, and sometimes impossible, to recall the whole array of available remedies so as to pick out the best . . . But a mere reminder is all he needs to make him at once master of the situation and enable him to prescribe exactly what his judgement tells him is needed for the occasion."

—*Merck's 1899 Manual*

Over one hundred years later, the information we need to carry with us has grown exponentially but our memories remain treacherous. In recent years, there has been a virtual explosion of clinical pathways and guidelines relating to treatment of a wide array of common medical conditions. Regrettably, many of these guidelines are not widely disseminated and we may be unaware of their existence. Moreover, these established pathways are not available at the time of the patient encounter, when on the spot decisions are necessary.

We developed *The Pocket Doctor* as a manual of instantly accessible therapeutic algorithms for common medical conditions based on many of these published clinical guidelines and pathways. Where such pathways may not exist, we have asked our expert authors to devise logical therapeutic strategies based on reliable medical literature as well as their specialized knowledge and experience. Authors have been given the latitude to update published guidelines when, in their opinion, valuable new therapies or drugs have emerged. We have also included a number of helpful tables, which have useful applications in clinical practice.

We have designed this book as a practical guide to patient management. We also believe it will be a valuable teaching aid, as the algorithms present a logical approach to the diagnosis and treatment of a broad range of medical problems. Most of our algorithms and tables have pertinent up-to-date references, which can be used as a further resource. Annotations and added source material will be accessible on our web site, ***www.PocketDoctor.com.*** Our goal was to provide you, the clinician, with a tool to remind you of the latest guidelines and diagnostic algorithms. It is our hope that *The Pocket Doctor* will help you "master the situation" in your daily rounds.

In this, our second edition, we have addressed a number of requests and comments received through our web site. We now have an index. We have also added new algorithms on smoking cessation, preoperative evaluation, syncope, depression, meningitis, and peripheral arterial disease. The pharmacology section was moved to the back so the IV dosing tables and the drug dose adjustments for renal failure are easier to find.

We again wish to thank all of our authors for their efforts in writing, revising, and updating the chapters in this book. We would like to thank Jerry Newman, Joy Newman, and Niels Buessem for their continued support and assistance with the book, Teri Deakens for her unflagging enthusiasm for this project, and Lawrence Husick and Amy Guskin for their help with the web site, **www.pocketdoctor.com.** Thanks also go to our readers for their suggestions, comments and enthusiastic reception of the book. Special thanks go to our wives, Jennifer and Rebecca, and our children, Rachel, Rebecca, Jeffrey, and Jane, for tolerating and encouraging us during the creation of this project.

Michael S. Sherman M.D.
Edward S. Schulman M.D.
Philadelphia, PA

1a: Periodic Health Examination for the General Population

Screening

Intervention	Age 25-49	Age 50-64	Age ≥ 65
Blood pressure	Q 2 years if last BP < 140/85. Q 1 year if last diastolic was 85-89		
Height and weight	Optimal frequency not defined. Monitor for unintended weight gain/loss and for obesity. Obesity defined as BMI (weight in kg/height in meters) ≥ 27.8 for men and ≥ 27.3 for women		
Total blood cholesterol	Q 5 years (recommendations vary), starting at 35 for men or 45 for women.	Q 5 years (recommendations vary)	Insufficient evidence for routine screening; screen depending on risk.
Fecal occult blood test	For clinical indications	Annual	Annual
Sigmoidoscopy	For clinical indications	USPSTF: Insufficient evidence for recommendation ACS: Q 3-5 years ACP: Q 10 years	USPSTF: Insufficient evidence for recommendation ACS: Q 3-5 years ACP: Q 10 years until age 70
Mammogram	USPSTF: Insufficient evidence for recommendation ACS, ACP: Q 1-2 years after age 40	USPSTF: Q 1-2 years ACP, ACS: Annual	USPSTF: Q 1-2 years until age 69 ACP: Annual until age 74
Breast examination	USPSTF: Insufficient evidence for recommendation ACS, ACP: Annual	Annual	USPSTF: Annual until age 70. Screening in older women should be considered on an individual basis.
Pap test	At onset of sexual activity and then Q 3 years	Q 3 years	Q 3 years; consider discontinuing if prior smears are consistently normal
Rubella serology or vaccination history	All women of childbearing potential	Not indicated	Not indicated
Prostate specific antigen (PSA) and digital exam of prostate	For clinical indications	USPSTF: Routine screening is not recommended ACP: Physicians should discuss and individualize decision to screen based on assessment of risk/benefit to the patient (age 50 – 69).	
TSH	For clinical indications	Once (esp females), then as indicated	For clinical indications

Counselling

Intervention	Age 25-49	Age 50-64	Age ≥ 65
Tobacco cessation	Each visit. Prescription of nicotine replacement therapy recommended as adjunct to counselling. See _Smoking Cessation_		
Assess for problem drinking	All adults and adolescents - careful history and/or standardized questionnaire. Pregnant women should be advised to abstain from alcohol during pregnancy. Counsel to avoid alcohol/drug use while driving, swimming, boating, etc.		
Dietary counselling:	Limit fat to < 30% of total calories and saturated fat to < 10 % of total calories. Limit cholesterol to < 300 mg/d. Emphasize foods containing fiber (fruits, whole grains, vegetables), lean meats, fish, poultry without skin, and low fat dairy products.		
Dietary calcium (women) (Consider adding Vitamin D3 800 U/d if post menopausal. See _Osteoporosis_)	1,000 mg/day 1,200 - 1,500 mg/d if pregnant or nursing	1,000 - 1,500 mg/day	1,000 - 1,500 mg/day

Recommendations are for general population not at high risk. Screening and interventions will differ for patients in high risk groups (for HIV, see _Prophylactic therapies for HIV Infection_). Except where noted, recommendations are from the Report of the U.S. Preventive Services Task Force (USPSTF). Other organizations may have different recommendations, some of which are noted above. ACP - American College of Physicians. ACS - American Cancer Society.

U.S. Preventive Services Task Force. Guide to clinical preventive services, 2nd ed. Baltimore: William & Wilkins, 1996 (http://158.72.20.10/pubs/guidecps/)

1b: Recommendations for routine vaccinations and post-exposure prophylaxis in adults

Vaccinations

Vaccine	Age 25-49	Age 50-64	Age ≥ 65
Influenza vaccine	Health care providers, residents of chronic care facilities, patients with chronic cardio-pulmonary disorders, diabetes, immunosuppression, renal dysfunction, and metabolic diseases should be vaccinated.		All persons
Tetanus vaccine series	All patients who have not received the primary tetanus series. Dose: 0, 2, and 8-14 months.		
Tetanus booster	Optimal frequency not established. Q 15-30 years felt to be adequate. Q 10 years for international travelers.		
Pneumococcal vaccine	Persons at high risk: cardiopulmonary disease, diabetes, asplenia, high exposure, immunocompromise	Persons at high risk, institutionalized patients	All persons
Hepatitis B	All young adults; susceptible adults in high risk groups including health care workers, homosexual men, IV drug users and their sex partners, persons with multiple sex partners, hemodialysis patients, blood product recipients. Dose: 10 or 20 μg (depending on product) IM at 0, 1 and 6 months. Check antibody response in patients with immunodeficiency.		
MMR vaccine	All persons born after 1956 without immunity (no prior vaccination, and no prior infection by history or serology)	Not indicated	Not indicated
Hepatitis A (HAV)	Travelers to endemic areas, homosexual men, IV drug users, military personnel, workers exposed to HAV, patients with chronic liver failure, patients who require clotting factor concentrates. Consider in residents / workers of institutions. Dose: 1,440 U at 0 and 6 to 12 months.		
Varicella	Healthy adults with no h/o varicella or prior vaccination and negative serology. Vaccination should be targeted to population at risk: health care workers, family contacts of immunosuppressed patients, day care centers, other institutions		
Lyme	Consider for persons engaging in activities that result in frequent or prolonged exposure to tick-infested habitat. May be considered for lesser exposure. Vaccination benefit beyond that provided by basic personal protection and early diagnosis and treatment of infection is uncertain.		

Post exposure prophylaxis

Exposure	Prophylaxis
Hepatitis A	Immune globulin 0.02 ml/kg IM within 2 weeks of exposure. Indicated for sexual contacts, close household contacts, staff and children at day care centers, staff and patients of custodial institutions, and food handlers exposed to a patient with Hepatitis A.
Hepatitis B	Unvaccinated exposed person: HBsAg + source: Hepatitis B Immunoglobulin (HBIG) 0.06 ml/kg IM. Initiate hepatitis B vaccination series within 7 days Unknown source: Initiate hepatitis B vaccination series within 7 days of exposure Previously vaccinated exposed person: Test exposed person for anti HBs. If < 10 SRU by RIA or negative ELISA, HBIG 0.06 ml/kg IM immediately plus HB Vaccine booster or (if vaccine refused) HBIG 0.06 ml/kg IM immediately and repeat at 1 month.
Meningococcus	Rifampin 600 mg BID X 2 days (contraindicated in pregnancy) OR Ofloxacin 400 mg (single dose; safety in pregnancy not established) Indicated for household or day care contacts, direct exposure to oral secretions of patient with meningococcal infection
Tetanus	Clean minor uncontaminated wounds: 0.5 ml tetanus toxoid IM if incomplete primary vaccination series or > 10 years from last tetanus booster. Serious and or contaminated wounds: 0.5 ml tetanus toxoid IM if > 5 years from last tetanus booster. Add human tetanus immune globulin if patient has not completed primary series.
HIV	See *HIV post-exposure prophylaxis*

U.S. Preventive Services Task Force. Guide to clinical preventive services, 2nd ed. Baltimore: William & Wilkins, 1996(http://text.nlm.nih.gov)

1c: Osteoporosis

History: Evaluate for risk factors
- Thin Caucasian or Asian female, non-exercising with a low calcium intake
- Early menopause (before age 45)
- 1.5 inches loss of height
- Low body weight post-menopause
- Family h/o osteoporosis and fracture
- Previous or current bone fracture
- Secondary causes: drugs (e.g. glucocorticoids, phenytoin, alcohol, tobacco), malignancy, hyperparathyroidism, hyperthyroidism, Cushing's disease, chronic liver or renal disease, hypogonadism, rheumatoid arthritis, organ transplantation, malabsorption syndromes, etc.

Biochemical testing to exclude secondary causes:
- Blood: CBC, BUN/Creat, serum Ca, TSH, LFTs, 25 hydroxy vitamin D (if age over 70), 1,25 vitamin D if impaired renal function
- 24 hr urinary calcium (Urinary marker of bone resorption?)
- ✓ testosterone level in hypogonadic male

- All patients should receive 1-1.5 g elemental calcium daily and Vitamin D (400 – 800 IU/d) if at risk for deficiency. Weight bearing exercises 3-5 X per week
- Check bone mineral density (BMD) measurements if any of above risk factors are present, or patient above 65 years of age without risk factors. Treat based on T score

T score (minus) –1 to –2.5
Osteopenia
1. Modify risk factors, e.g. cigarette smoking, excess alcohol.
2. 0.625 mg conjugated estrogen or equivalent with or without progesterone cyclically or continuous

OR

3. Bisphosphonate (e.g. Alendronate 10 mg qd or 70 mg q week, or Risendronate 5 mg/d if estrogen not applicable)

OR

4. SERM (selective estrogen receptor modulator) e.g. Raloxifene 60 mg/d if estrogen not applicable

OR

5. Calcitonin 200 IU/d intranasal or SC if above not suitable

T score lower than (minus) –2.5
Osteoporosis
1. Modify risk factors, e.g. cigarette smoking, excess alcohol.
2. Bisphosphonate (e.g. Alendronate 10 mg/d or 70 mg q week, OR Risendronate 5 mg/d) as "first line" therapy

OR

3. 0.625 mg conjugated estrogen or equivalent with or without progesterone cyclically or continuous

OR

4. SERM (selective estrogen receptor modulator) e.g. Raloxifene 60 mg/d if estrogen not applicable

OR

5. Calcitonin 200 IU/d intranasal or SC provided no osteoporosis of the hip is present
6. If hypogonadic male, consider replacing testosterone (controversial)

Repeat BMD at ± 1.5 years after starting Rx to reassess progress

Eastell R. Treatment of postmenopausal osteoporosis. N Engl J Med 338: 736-746, 1998
NOF guidelines. Osteoporosis International 1998 Suppl 4: S1-S88

1d: Preoperative Evaluation of the Patient Undergoing Noncardiac Surgery

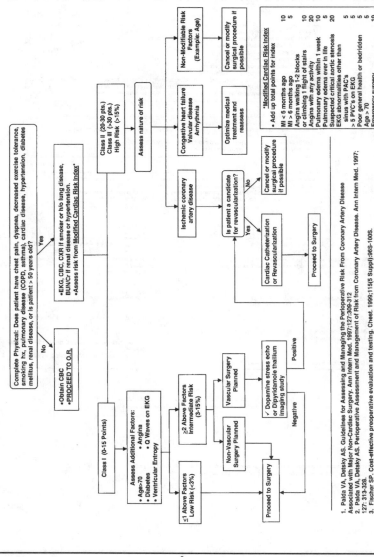

Complete Physical: Does patient have chest pain, dyspnea, decreased exercise tolerance, smoking hx, pulmonary disease (COPD, asthma), cardiac disease, hypertension, diabetes mellitus, renal disease, or is patient > 50 years old?

No
- Obtain CBC
- **PROCEED TO O.R.**

Yes
- EKG, CBC, CXR if lung disease, BUN/Cr if renal disease or hypertension.
- Assess risk from *Modified Cardiac Risk Index*

Class I (0-15 Points)

Assess Additional Factors:
- Age>70
- Angina
- Diabetes
- Q Waves on EKG
- Ventricular Entropy

≥2 Above Factors Intermediate Risk (3-15%)

≤1 Above Factors Low Risk (<3%)

Vascular Surgery Planned

Non-Vascular Surgery Planned

✓ Dopamine stress echo or Dipyridamole thallium imaging study

Positive

Negative

Proceed to Surgery

Class II (20-30 pts.) Class III (>30 pts.) High Risk (>15%)

Assess nature of risk

Ischemic coronary artery disease

Congestive heart failure Valvular disease Arrhythmia

Optimize medical treatment and reasses

Non-Modifiable Risk Factors (Example: Age)

Cancel or modify surgical procedure if possible

Is patient a candidate for revascularization?

No
Cancel or modify surgical procedure if possible

Yes
Cardiac Catheterization or Revascularization

Proceed to Surgery

Modified Cardiac Risk Index
- Add up total points for index

MI < 6 months ago	10
MI > 6 months ago	5
Angina walking 1-2 blocks or climbing 1 flight of stairs	10
Angina with any activity	20
Pulmonary edema within 1 week	10
Pulmonary edema ever in life	5
Suspected critical aortic stenosis	20
EKG abnormalities other than sinus with PAC's	5
> 5 PVC's on EKG	5
Poor general health or bedridden	5
Age >70	5
Emergency surgery	10
Total:	

1. Palda VA, Detsky AS. Guidelines for Assessing and Managing the Perioperative Risk From Coronary Artery Disease Associated with Major Non-Cardiac Surgery. Ann Intern Med. 1997;127:309-312
2. Palda VA, Detsky AS. Perioperative Assessment and Management of Risk from Coronary Artery Disease. Ann Intern Med. 1997; 127: 313-326.
3. Fischer SP. Cost-effective preoperative evaluation and testing. Chest. 1999;115(5 Suppl):965-100S.

1e: Smoking Cessation

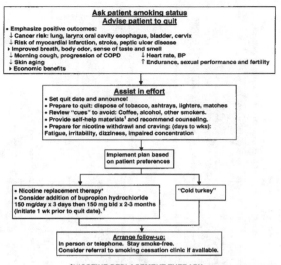

Ask patient smoking status
Advise patient to quit
- Emphasize positive outcomes:
  ↓ Cancer risk: lung, larynx oral cavity esophagus, bladder, cervix
  ↓ Risk of myocardial infarction, stroke, peptic ulcer disease
- ► Improved breath, body odor, sense of taste and smell
  ↓ Morning cough, progression of COPD   ↓ Heart rate, BP
  ↓ Skin aging   ↑ Endurance, sexual performance and fertility
  ► Economic benefits

Assist in effort
- Set quit date and announce!
- Prepare to quit: dispose of tobacco, ashtrays, lighters, matches
- Review "cues" to avoid: Coffee, alcohol, other smokers.
- Provide self-help materials† and recommend counseling.
- Prepare for nicotine withdrawl and craving: (days to wks):
  Fatigue, irritability, dizziness, impaired concentration

Implement plan based on patient preferences

- Nicotine replacement therapy*
- Consider addition of bupropion hydrochloride 150 mg/day x 3 days then 150 mg bid x 2-3 months (initiate 1 wk prior to quit date). ‡

"Cold turkey"

Arrange follow-up:
In person or telephone. Stay smoke-free.
Consider referral to smoking cessation clinic if available.

*NICOTINE REPLACEMENT THERAPY

PRODUCT	ABSORPTION	DOSAGE	DURATION	CONSIDERATIONS
Nicotine Patch	Slow	1 patch per day. ↓ dosage slowly; change site daily	6-10 weeks	Caution in pregnancy and within 4 weeks of MI. Apply on relatively hairless area between head and waste
Nicoderm CQ® (OTC) and Habitrol® (Rx required)		21 mg/24 hr 14 mg/24 hr 7 mg/24 hr	4-6 weeks 2 weeks 2 weeks	
Nicotrol® (OTC)	Slow	15 mg/16 hr	6 weeks	
Prostep ® (Rx required)		22 mg/24 hr 11 mg/24 hr	4-8 weeks 2-4 weeks (optional)	
Nicotine Nasal Spray Nicotrol NS® (Rx) (Dispensed in 10 ml metered spray pump)	Fastest delivery. Satisfies immediate craving	0.5 mg/ dose 1-2x/hr or prn. Deep breath, spray then exhale. Do not sniff.		Can use prn for urge to smoke in combination with patch. Nose and eye irritation
Nicotine "gum" Nicotine polacriiex (Nicorette®) (OTC)	Faster than patch. Frequent use required. Cannot eat or drink while gum in mouth	2 mg, 4 mg; ≥9 pieces/day. Discard after 30 minutes. Also, can use prn for urge to smoke even with patch	≤ 3 months	Chew to peppery taste and tingle, then park between cheek and gum. Repeat as needed.
Nicotine oral inhaler Nicotrol inhaler (Rx)	Faster than patches. Nicotine vapor is not inhaled – is absorbed through the oral cavity	0.1 mg/cartridge 80 puffs over 20 min. ≥6 cartridges/day	3-6 weeks	Shaped like a cigarette. Mimics "hand to mouth" and puffing on a cigarette

† Materials include Freedom From Smoking® guidebooks, video- and audio tapes. Available from http://www.lungsusa.org/.
‡Contraindicated in patients with history of eating disorders, alcohol abuse, head trauma and seizures

1. West R et al. Smoking cessation guidelines for health professionals: an update. Thorax 2000; 55: 987-99
2. Smoking Cessation: Clinical Practice Guideline (No. 18). Rockville, Md: US Dept of Health and Human Services, Public Health Service, Agency for Health Care Policy and Research, Centers for DiseaseControl and Prevention; 1996. DHHS Publication No. (AHCPR) 96-0892.
3. Jorenby DE, et al. A controlled trial of sustained-release buprorion, a nicotine patch, or both for smoking cessation. N Engl J Med. 1999;340:685-691

1f: Prophylaxis for Deep Venous Thrombosis

Condition	Incidence of DVT	Options for DVT prophylaxis
General surgery	20-25%	• Low dose heparin 5,000 U SC Q8 or Q12H. Begin 2 hours pre-op, continue until discharge • Enoxaparin 40 mg SC QD; begin postoperatively (post op) • Dalteparin 5,000 U SC QD; begin 1-2h preoperatively (pre op). • Extrinsic pneumatic compression (EPC) sleeves[1] • Dextran: 500 cc upon initiation of surgery, 500 cc post op over 12-18 hours, then 500 cc daily over 24 hours for 3-5 days. (some clinicians prefer to give 10cc/kg during surgery and 7.5 cc/kg daily postoperatively)
Multiple trauma		Enoxaparin 30 mg q12h
Total hip replacement (THR) or hip fracture	45-57% 36-60%	• Enoxaparin 30 mg q12h starting 12-24 h post op or 40 mg qd starting 10-12 h pre-op • Dalteparin 5,000 units qd starting 1 hr pre op (THR indication only) • Danaparoid 750 U 1-2h pre op, then q12h • Warfarin[1] 10 mg evening before surgery, then 5 mg evening of surgery: maintain INR of 2-3 until discharge • Adjusted dose heparin: 3,600 U q8h post op, adjust by 500 U increments to maintain PTT at top normal value. May add EPC sleeves as adjuvant Rx[1]
Total knee replacement	40-80%	• Enoxaparin 30 mg q12h starting 12-24 h post op or 40 mg qd starting 10-12 h pre-op • Ardeparin 50 U/kg q12h starting 12-24 h post op May add EPC sleeves as adjuvant Rx[1]
Craniotomy	18-43%	• EPC sleeves[1] • Low dose heparin 5,000 U SC Q8 or Q12H
Acute spinal cord injury	49-72%	• Adjusted dose heparin: 3,500 U given q8h, adjust by 500 U increments to maintain PTT at top normal value. • Enoxaparin 30 mg q12h • Warfarin[1] may be effective (INR 2-3) • Low dose heparin plus elastic stockings plus EPC sleeves[1] may have benefit when used together
Spinal cord surgery	(high)	EPC sleeves plus low dose heparin or EPC sleeves alone[1]
Gynecologic surgery	Nonmalignancy surgery: Abdominal hysterectomy: 12-15% Vaginal hysterectomy: 6-7% Malignancy surgery: Abdominal hysterectomy: 35%	• Low dose heparin 5,000 U SC Q8 or Q12H. Begin 2 hours pre-op, continue until discharge • Enoxaparin 30 mg q12h starting 12-24 h post op or 40 mg qd starting 10-12 h pre-op • Dalteparin 5,000 U SC QD; begin 10-12h preop • EPC sleeves[1] or • Dextran. Use as for general surgery above.
Urologic surgery	Open prostatectomy: 20-50% TURP: 7-10%	• Low dose heparin 5,000 U SC Q8 or Q12H. Begin 2 hours pre-op, continue until discharge • Enoxaparin 30 mg q12h starting 12-24 h post op or 40 mg qd starting 10-12 h pre-op • Dalteparin 5,000 U SC QD; begin 10-12h preop • EPC sleeves[1]
General medical patients with clinical risk factors for thromboembolism		• Low dose heparin 5,000 U SC Q8 or Q12H • Enoxaparin 40 mg SC qd • Danaparoid 750 U q12h (if unable to take heparin or enoxaparin) • EPC sleeves[1]
Myocardial infarction		• Heparin (prophylactic low dose or full dose as clinically indicated) • Enoxaparin 40 mg SC qd • EPC sleeves when heparin is contraindicated[1]

1. Place sleeves prior to surgery (if applicable). Sleeves must be worn continuously for 48-72 hours. After 48-72 hours, consider pharmacologic Rx. Patients immobilized >72 hours without prophylaxis must have screening for DVT prior to placing the EPC sleeves
2. Do not give warfarin to pregnant patients. Modified warfarin method: 10 mg the evening of surgery; skip post op day 1; adjust daily INR to 2-3; continue to discharge

1. Goldhaber S, Morpurgo M for the WHO/ISFC Task Force on Pulmonary Embolism. Diagnosis, treatment and prevention of pulmonary embolism. JAMA 268: 1727-1733, 1992
2. Fifth ACCP consensus conference on antithrombotic therapy. Chest 114 (suppl): 531S-560S, 1998
3. Merli G. Prophylaxis for deep venous thrombosis and pulmonary embolism in the surgical patient. In Merli G, Weitz H, eds. Medical management of the surgical patient, 2nd ed. WB Saunders Co., Philadelphia, 1998

1g: Treatment of Hypercholesterolemia

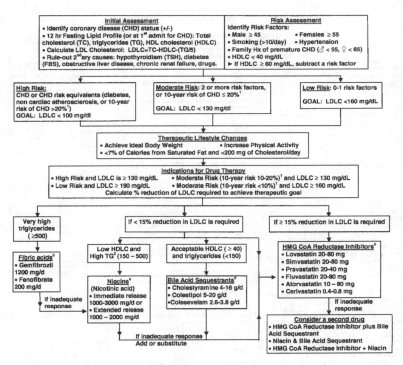

Initial Assessment
- Identify coronary disease (CHD) status (+/-)
- 12 hr Fasting Lipid Profile (or at 1st admit for CHD): Total cholesterol (TC), triglycerides (TG), HDL cholesterol (HDLC)
- Calculate LDL Cholesterol: LDLC=TC-HDLC-(TG/5)
- Rule-out 2nd ary causes: hypothyroidism (TSH), diabetes (FBS), obstructive liver disease, chronic renal failure, drugs.

Risk Assessment
Identify Risk Factors:
- Male ≥ 45   • Females ≥ 55
- Smoking (>10/day)   • Hypertension
- Family Hx of premature CHD (♂ < 55, ♀ < 65)
- HDLC < 40 mg/dL
► If HDLC ≥ 60 mg/dL, subtract a risk factor

High Risk:
CHD or CHD risk equivalents (diabetes, non cardiac atherosclerosis, or 10-year risk of CHD >20%[1])
GOAL: LDLC < 100 mg/dl

Moderate Risk: 2 or more risk factors, or 10-year risk of CHD ≤ 20%[1]
GOAL: LDLC < 130 mg/dl

Low Risk: 0-1 risk factors
GOAL: LDLC <160 mg/dL

Therapeutic Lifestyle Changes
- Achieve ideal Body Weight   • Increase Physical Activity
- <7% of Calories from Saturated Fat and <200 mg of Cholesterol/day

Indications for Drug Therapy
- High Risk and LDLC is ≥ 130 mg/dL   • Moderate Risk (10-year risk 10-20%)[1] and LDLC ≥ 130 mg/dL
- Low Risk and LDLC ≥ 190 mg/dL   • Moderate Risk (10-year risk <10%)[1] and LDLC ≥ 160 mg/dL
Calculate % reduction of LDLC required to achieve therapeutic goal

Very high triglycerides (≥500)

Fibric acids[3]
- Gemfibrozil 1200 mg/d
- Fenofibrate 200 mg/d

If inadequate response

If < 15% reduction in LDLC is required

Low HDLC and High TG[2] (150 – 500)

Niacins[4]
(Nicotinic acid)
- Immediate release 1000-3000 mg/d or
- Extended release 1000 – 2000 mg/d

If inadequate response
Add or substitute

Acceptable HDLC (≥ 40) and triglycerides (<150)

Bile Acid Sequestrants[5]
- Cholestyramine 4-16 g/d
- Colestipol 5-20 g/d
- Colesevelam 2.6-3.8 g/d

If ≥ 15% reduction in LDLC is required

HMG CoA Reductase Inhibitors[6]
- Lovastatin 20-80 mg
- Simvastatin 20-80 mg
- Pravastatin 20-40 mg
- Fluvastatin 20-80 mg
- Atorvastatin 10 – 80 mg
- Cerivastatin 0.4-0.8 mg

If inadequate response

Consider a second drug
- HMG CoA Reductase Inhibitor plus Bile Acid Sequestrant
- Niacin & Bile Acid Sequestrant
- HMG CoA Reductase Inhibitor + Niacin

2. Metabolic Syndrome = 3 or more of the following: Abdominal obesity, High Triglycerides, Low HDLC, BP ≥130/85, FBS ≥ 100 mg/dL. May need to use non-HDLC (TC-HDLC) as a goal level. Non-HDLC goal levels = LDL goal levels+30 mg/dL.
3. Effective in lowering triglycerides and raising HDLC, but minimal LDLC reduction (10-15%). Small risk of liver function abnormalities or myopathy, especially when added to a statin
4. Lowers triglycerides, LDLC (10-25%); raises HDLC, but causes flushing, hyperglycemia, pruritus, hyperuricemia, and dose-related hepatotoxicity.
5. Good efficacy and safety record and can be used in pre-menopausal women but only 10-30% LDLC reduction.
6. Highly effective (20-60% ↓ in LDLC); not recommended for women of childbearing potential. Small risk of myopathy. Follow liver function tests.

1. Estimate of 10 year risk for coronary heart disease: add the sum of all point scores based on age and sex:

Sex	20-34		35-39		40-44		45-49		50-54		55-59		60-64		65-69		70-74		75-79	
	m	f	m	f	m	f	m	f	m	f	m	f	m	f	m	f	m	f	m	f
Age	-9	-7	-4	-3	0	0	3	3	6	6	8	8	8	1 1	1 1	1 1	1 2	1 2	1 4	1 3
													0	0	1	2	2	4	3	6
TC <160	0	0	0	0	0	0	0	0	0	0	0	0	0	0	0	0	0	0	0	0
TC 160-199	4	4	4	4	3	3	3	3	2	2	2	2	1	1	1	1	0	1	0	1
TC 200-239	7	8	7	8	5	6	5	6	3	4	3	4	1	2	1	2	0	1	0	1
TC 240-279	9	11	9	11	6	8	6	8	4	5	4	5	2	3	2	3	1	2	1	2
TC >279	1 1	13	11	13	8	10	8	1 0	5	7	5	7	3	4	3	4	1	2	1	2

Point total	Risk: males
<5	≤ 1%
5-6	2%
7-9	3-5%
10	6%
11	8%
12	10%
13	12%
14	16%
15	20%
16	25%
≥17	>30%

Point total	Risk: female
<12	≤ 1%
13-14	2%
15-17	3-5%
18	6%
19	8%
20	11%
21	14%
22	17%
23	22%
24	27%
≥ 25	≥30%

Summary of the NCEP Adult Treatment Panel III Report. JAMA 285: 2486-2497, 2001

2a: Acute Myocardial Infarction

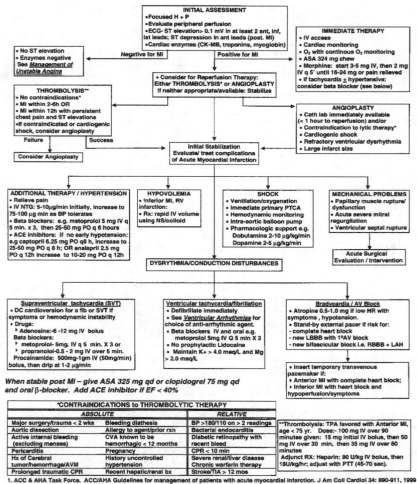

INITIAL ASSESSMENT
- Focused H + P
- Evaluate peripheral perfusion
- ECG- ST elevation> 0.1 mV in at least 2 ant, inf, lat leads; ST depression in ant leads (post. MI)
- Cardiac enzymes (CK-MB, troponins, myoglobin)

Negative for MI → Positive for MI

IMMEDIATE THERAPY
- IV access
- Cardiac monitoring
- O₂ with continous O₂ monitoring
- ASA 324 mg chew
- Morphine: start 3-5 mg IV, then 2 mg IV q 5' until 16-24 mg or pain relieved
- If tachycardia ± hypertensive: consider beta blocker (see below)

- No ST elevation
- Enzymes negative
See *Management of Unstable Angina*

- Consider for Reperfusion Therapy:
Either THROMBOLYSIS* or ANGIOPLASTY
If neither appropriate/available: Stabilize

THROMBOLYSIS**
- No contraindications*
- MI within 2-6h OR
- MI within 12h with persistent chest pain and ST elevations
- If contraindicated or cardiogenic shock, consider angioplasty

Failure / Success

Consider Angioplasty

ANGIOPLASTY
- Cath lab immediately available (< 1 hour to reperfusion) and/or
- Contraindication to lytic therapy*
- Cardiogenic shock
- Refractory ventricular dysrhythmia
- Large infarct size

Initial Stabilization
Evaluate/ treat complications
of Acute Myocardial Infarction

ADDITIONAL THERAPY / HYPERTENSION
- Relieve pain
- IV NTG: 5-10µg/min initially, increase to 75-100 µg min as BP tolerates
- Beta blockers: e.g. metoprolol 5 mg IV q 5 min. x 3, then 25-50 mg PO q 6 hours
- ACE inhibitors: if no early hypotension; e.g captopril 6.25 mg PO q8 h, increase to 25-50 mg PO q 8 h; OR enalapril 2.5 mg PO q 12h increase to 10-20 mg PO q 12h

HYPOVOLEMIA
- Inferior MI, RV infarction:
- Rx: rapid IV volume using NS/colloid

SHOCK
- Ventilation/oxygenation
- Immediate primary PTCA
- Hemodynamic monitoring
- Intra-aortic balloon pump
- Pharmacologic support e.g. Dobutamine 2-10 µg/kg/min Dopamine 2-5 µg/kg/min

MECHANICAL PROBLEMS
- Papillary muscle rupture/ dysfunction
- Acute severe mitral regurgitation
- Ventricular septal rupture

Acute Surgical Evaluation / Intervention

DYSRYTHMIA/CONDUCTION DISTURBANCES

Supraventricular tachycardia (SVT)
- DC cardioversion for a fib or SVT if symptoms or hemodynamic instability
- Drugs:
  - Adenosine:-6 -12 mg IV bolus
  Beta blockers:
  - metoprolol- 5mg. IV q 5 min. X 3 or
  - propranolol-0.5 - 2 mg IV over 5 min.
  Procainamide: 500mg-1gm IV (50mg/min) bolus, then drip at 1-2 µg/min

Ventricular tachycardia/fibrillation
- Defibrillate immediately
- See *Ventricular Arrhythmias* for choice of anti-arrhythmic agent.
- Beta blockers e.g. metoprolol 5mg IV Q 5 min X 3
- No prophylactic Lidocaine
- Maintain K+ > 4.0 meq/L and Mg > 2.0 meq/L

Bradycardia / AV Block
- Atropine 0.5-1.0 mg if low HR with symptoms , hypotension.
- Stand-by external pacer if risk for:
  - complete heart block
  - new LBBB with 1°AV block
  - new bifascicular block i.e. RBBB + LAH

- Insert temporary transvenous pacemaker if:
  - Anterior MI with complete heart block;
  - Inferior MI with heart block and hypoperfusion/symptoms

When stable post MI – give ASA 325 mg qd or clopidogrel 75 mg qd and oral β-blocker. Add ACE inhibitor if EF < 40%

*CONTRAINDICATIONS to THROMBOLYTIC THERAPY

ABSOLUTE		RELATIVE	
Major surgery/trauma < 2 wks	Bleeding diathesis	BP >180/110 on > 2 readings	
Aortic dissection	Allergy to agent/prior rxn	Bacterial endocarditis	
Active internal bleeding (excluding menses)	CVA known to be hemorrhagic < 12 months	Diabetic retinopathy with recent bleed	
Pericarditis	Pregnancy	CPR < 10 min	
Hx of Cerebral tumor/hemorrhage/AVM	History uncontrolled hypertension	Severe renal/liver disease Chronic warfarin therapy	
Prolonged traumatic CPR	Recent hepatic/renal bx	Stroke/TIA > 12 mos	

**Thrombolysis: TPA favored with Anterior MI, age < 75 yr. Dose:- 100 mg IV over 90 minutes given: 15 mg initial IV bolus, then 50 mg IV over 30 min, then 35 mg IV over 60 minutes
Adjunct RX: Heparin: 80 U/kg bolus, then 18U/kg/hr; adjust with PTT (45-70 sec).

1. ACC & AHA Task Force. ACC/AHA Guidelines for management of patients with acute myocardial infarction. J Am Coll Cardiol 34: 890-911, 1999
2. The GUSTO Investigators. An international randomized trial comparing four thrombolytic strategies for acute myocardial infarction. N Eng J Med 1993; 329:1615-1622.
3. Anderson, H.V., Willerson, J.E. Thrombolysis in acute myocardial infarction. N Eng J Med 1993;329:703-709.

2b: Management of Unstable Angina

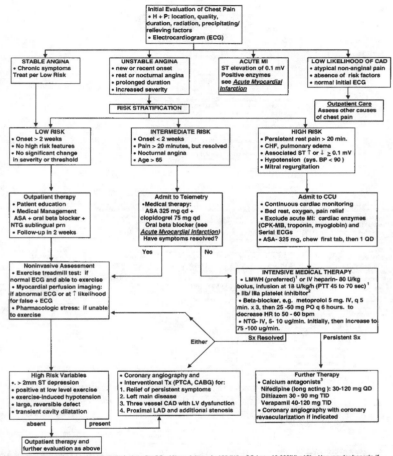

Initial Evaluation of Chest Pain
- H + P: location, quality, duration, radiation, precipitating/relieving factors
- Electrocardiogram (ECG)

STABLE ANGINA
- Chronic symptoms
Treat per Low Risk

UNSTABLE ANGINA
- new or recent onset
- rest or nocturnal angina
- prolonged duration
- increased severity

ACUTE MI
ST elevation of 0.1 mV
Positive enzymes
see *Acute Myocardial Infarction*

LOW LIKELIHOOD OF CAD
- atypical non-anginal pain
- absence of risk factors
- normal initial ECG

RISK STRATIFICATION

Outpatient Care
Assess other causes of chest pain

LOW RISK
- Onset > 2 weeks
- No high risk features
- No significant change in severity or threshold

INTERMEDIATE RISK
- Onset < 2 weeks
- Pain > 20 minutes, but resolved
- Nocturnal angina
- Age > 65

HIGH RISK
- Persistent rest pain > 20 min.
- CHF, pulmonary edema
- Associated ST ↑ or ↓ ≥ 0.1 mV
- Hypotension (sys. BP < 90)
- Mitral regurgitation

Outpatient therapy
- Patient education
- Medical Management
ASA + oral beta blocker + NTG sublingual prn
- Follow-up in 2 weeks

Admit to Telemetry
- Medical therapy:
ASA 325 mg qd + clopidogrel 75 mg qd
Oral beta blocker (see *Acute Myocardial Infarction*)
Have symptoms resolved?

Yes   No

Admit to CCU
- Continuous cardiac monitoring
- Bed rest, oxygen, pain relief
- Exclude acute MI: cardiac enzymes (CPK-MB, troponin, myoglobin) and Serial ECGs
- ASA- 325 mg, chew first tab, then 1 QD

Noninvasive Assessment
- Exercise treadmill test: if normal ECG and able to exercise
- Myocardial perfusion imaging: if abnormal ECG or at ↑ likelihood for false + ECG
- Pharmacologic stress: if unable to exercise

INTENSIVE MEDICAL THERAPY
- LMWH (preferred)[1] or IV heparin- 80 U/kg bolus, infusion at 18 U/kg/h (PTT 45 to 70 sec)[1]
- IIb/ IIIa platelet inhibitor[2]
- Beta-blocker, e.g. metoprolol 5 mg. IV, q 5 min. x 3, then 25 -50 mg PO q 6 hours. to decrease HR to 50 - 60 bpm
- NTG- IV, 5- 10 ug/min. initially, then increase to 75 -100 ug/min.

Either   Sx Resolved   Persistent Sx

High Risk Variables
- > 2mm ST depression
- positive at low level exercise
- exercise-induced hypotension
- large, reversible defect
- transient cavity dilatation

- Coronary angiography and
- Interventional Tx (PTCA, CABG) for:
1. Relief of persistent symptoms
2. Left main disease
3. Three vessel CAD with LV dysfunction
4. Proximal LAD and additional stenosis

Further Therapy
- Calcium antagonists[3]
Nifedipine (long acting): 30-120 mg QD
Diltiazem 30 - 90 mg TID
Verapamil 40-120 mg TID
- Coronary angiography with coronary revascularization if indicated

absent   present

Outpatient therapy and further evaluation as above

1. Low molecular weight heparin: enoxaparin 1 mg/kg SC q12h or dalteparin 120 IU/kg SC (max 10,000IU) q12h. Use regular heparin if creatinine clearance <30 ml/min.
2. Abciximab 0.25 mg/kg bolus, then 10 µg/min, or eptifibatide 180 µg/kg, then 2 µg/kg/min, or tirofiban 0.4 µg/kg/min X 30', then 0.1 µg/kg/min (adjust for weight and creatinine)
3. Calcium antagonists are 2nd line therapy to be used only if symptoms persist despite β-blocker, Nitrates, ASA and heparin. Use with extreme caution in patients with LV dysfunction. PTCA – coronary angioplasty. CAD – coronary artery disease

Braunwald E et al. Unstable Angina: Diagnosis and Management. CPG # 10 AHCPR No 94-0602. Rockville, MD, 1994
McClellan JR. Unstable Angina: Prognosis, Noninvasive Risk Assessment and Strategies for Management. Clin Cardiol 1994; 17:229-238
Girl S, Waters DD. Pathophysiology and Initial Management of the Acute Coronary Syndromes. Curr Opin Cardiol 1996; 11:394-402.
Lincoff AM et al. Platelet glycoprotein IIb/IIIa receptor blockade in coronary artery disease. J Am Coll Cardiol 2000; 35(5):1103-15

2c: Congestive Heart Failure

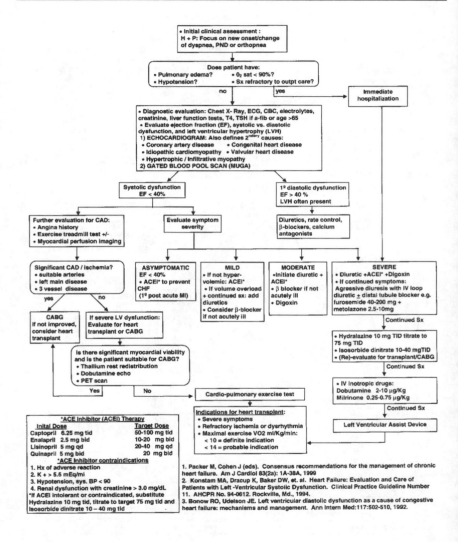

2d: Evaluation of the Patient with Syncope

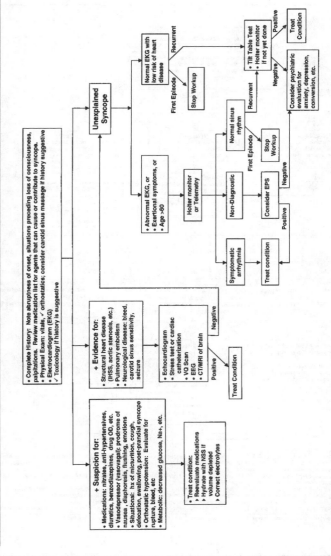

EPS-Electrophysiologic study; VQ- Ventilation/perfusion scan; MRI-Magnetic Resonance Imaging; CT-Computerized Tomography; EEG-Electroencephalogram; NSS-0.9% Saline Solution; IHSS-Idiopathic hypertrophic subaortic stenosis

Linzer M, Yang EH, Estes NAM, et al. Diagnosing Syncope. Part 1: Value of History, Physical Examination and Electrocardiography. Ann Intern Med. 1997; 126: 989-996.
Linzer M, Yang EH, Estes NAM, et al. Diagnosing Syncope. Part 2: Unexplained Syncope. Ann Intern Med. 1997; 127: 76-86.

2e: Narrow Complex Tachycardia

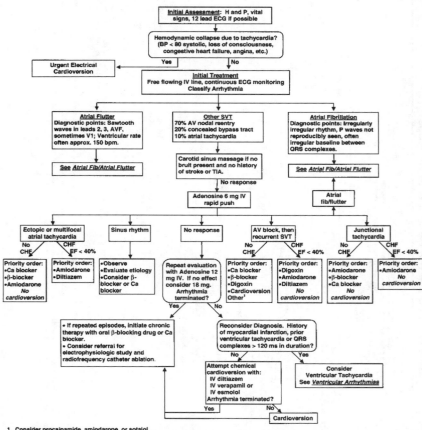

1. Consider procainamide, amiodarone, or sotalol

Cardioversion:	Synchronized – 100 joules. Use 200, 300 and 360 joules (monophasic waveform) if needed. Use adequate sedation or anesthesia.
IV Adenosine:	6 mg IV by rapid push. If no effect use 12 mg. Higher doses rarely necessary. Adenosine may induce atrial fibrillation. Use 3 mg initial dose if patient taking dipyridamole.
IV Amiodarone:	150 mg bolus over 10 min, repeat q10-15' prn. Max dose: 2.2 g/24h. Maintenance: 1 mg/min for 6 hours, 0.5 mg/min thereafter
Ca blocker:	Calcium channel blocker (diltiazem, verapamil)
IV Digoxin:	0.125 - 0.5 mg IV loading dose, up to 0.75 to 1.25 mg in 24 hours in divided doses, 0.125 - 0.375 mg daily maintenance dose.
IV Diltiazem:	Loading Dose 10 - 25 mg IV slow push, followed by 5 - 15 mg/min maintenance infusion. Causes hypotension.
IV Esmolol:	500 mcg/kg/min for 1 min loading dose, followed by 50 - 200 mcg/kg/min maintenance infusion. Causes hypotension.
IV Verapamil:	2.5 - 5 mg IV slow push. May repeat up to 15 - 20 mg total. Never use if ventricular tachycardia suspected. Causes hypotension.

Guidelines 2000 for Cardiopulmonary Resuscitation and Emergency Cardiac Care. Circulation; 2000; 102 (suppl I): I-158-165.

2f: Atrial Fibrillation/Atrial Flutter

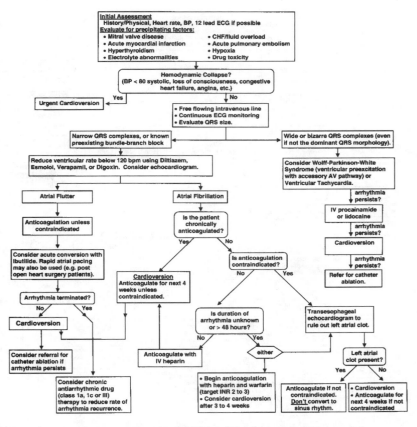

Initial Assessment
History/Physical, Heart rate, BP, 12 lead ECG if possible
Evaluate for precipitating factors:
- Mitral valve disease
- Acute myocardial infarction
- Hyperthyroidism
- Electrolyte abnormalities
- CHF/fluid overload
- Acute pulmonary embolism
- Hypoxia
- Drug toxicity

Hemodynamic Collapse?
(BP < 80 systolic, loss of consciousness, congestive heart failure, angina, etc.)

Yes → **Urgent Cardioversion**

No →
- Free flowing intravenous line
- Continuous ECG monitoring
- Evaluate QRS size.

Narrow QRS complexes, or known preexisting bundle-branch block

Reduce ventricular rate below 120 bpm using Diltiazem, Esmolol, Verapamil, or Digoxin. Consider echocardiogram.

Atrial Flutter

Anticoagulation unless contraindicated

Consider acute conversion with Ibutilide. Rapid atrial pacing may also be used (e.g. post open heart surgery patients).

Arrhythmia terminated?

No → **Cardioversion**
Yes →

Consider referral for catheter ablation if arrhythmia persists

Consider chronic antiarrhythmic drug (class 1a, 1c or III) therapy to reduce rate of arrhythmia recurrence.

Atrial Fibrillation

Is the patient chronically anticoagulated?

Yes → Cardioversion. Anticoagulate for next 4 weeks unless contraindicated.

No → Is anticoagulation contraindicated?

No → Is duration of arrhythmia unknown or > 48 hours?

No → Anticoagulate with IV heparin

Yes → either

- Begin anticoagulation with heparin and warfarin (target INR 2 to 3)
- Consider cardioversion after 3 to 4 weeks

Yes → Transesophageal echocardiogram to rule out left atrial clot.

Left atrial clot present?

Yes → Anticoagulate if not contraindicated. **Don't** convert to sinus rhythm.

No →
- Cardioversion
- Anticoagulate for next 4 weeks if not contraindicated

Wide or bizarre QRS complexes (even if not the dominant QRS morphology).

Consider Wolff-Parkinson-White Syndrome (ventricular preexcitation with accessory AV pathway) or Ventricular Tachycardia.

arrhythmia persists?

IV procainamide or lidocaine

arrhythmia persists?

Cardioversion

arrhythmia persists?

Refer for catheter ablation.

Cardioversion: Synchronized with 100 Joules. Use 200, 300 and 360 Joules if necessary. Ensure adequate sedation or anesthesia.
IV Ibutilide: 1 mg IV over 10 mins. Wait 10 mins, if no effect, may repeat dose once. May induce ventricular tachycardia (Torsades de pointes).
IV Digoxin: 0.125 - 0.5 mg IV loading dose, up to 0.75 to 1.25 mg over 24 hours in divided doses, 0.125 - 0.375 mg daily maintenance dose.
IV Diltiazem: Loading Dose 10 - 25 mg IV slow push, followed by 5 - 15 mg/min maintenance infusion. Produces hypotension.
IV Esmolol: 500 mcg/kg/min for 1 min loading dose, followed by 50 - 200 mcg/kg/min maintenance infusion. Produces hypotension.
IV Verapamil: 2.5 - 5 mg IV slow push. May repeat up to 15 - 20 mg total dose. Never use if ventricular tachycardia suspected.
IV Procainamide: 15 mg/kg IV at 25 mg/min maximum rate loading dose; 1 - 4 mg/min maintenance infusion. Produces hypotension.

Circulation, 2000; 102 (suppl I): I-158-165.
Prystowsky EN, Benson DW, Fuster V, et al: Management of Patients with Atrial Fibrillation. AHA Medical/Scientific Statement. Circulation 1996;93:1262-77.

2g: AV block

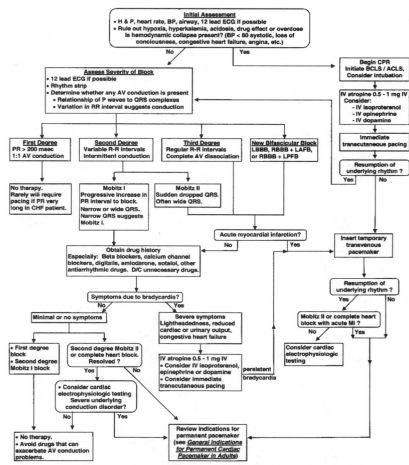

Initial Assessment
- H & P, heart rate, BP, airway, 12 lead ECG if possible
- Rule out hypoxia, hyperkalemia, acidosis, drug effect or overdose
  Is hemodynamic collapse present? (BP < 80 systolic, loss of conciousness, congestive heart failure, angina, etc.)

No / Yes

Begin CPR
Initiate BCLS / ACLS, Consider intubation

IV atropine 0.5 - 1 mg IV
Consider:
- IV isoproterenol
- IV epinephrine
- IV dopamine

Immediate transcutaneous pacing

Resumption of underlying rhythm ?
Yes | No

Assess Severity of Block
- 12 lead ECG if possible
- Rhythm strip
- Determine whether any AV conduction is present
  - Relationship of P waves to QRS complexes
  - Variation in RR interval suggests conduction

First Degree
PR > 200 msec
1:1 AV conduction

Second Degree
Variable R-R intervals
Intermittent conduction

Third Degree
Regular R-R intervals
Complete AV dissociation

New Bifascicular Block
LBBB, RBBB + LAFB, or RBBB + LPFB

No therapy.
Rarely will require pacing if PR very long in CHF patient.

Mobitz I
Progressive increase in PR interval to block. Narrow or wide QRS. Narrow QRS suggests Mobitz I.

Mobitz II
Sudden dropped QRS. Often wide QRS.

Acute myocardial infarction?
No | Yes

Insert temporary transvenous pacemaker

Resumption of underlying rhythm ?
Yes | No

Obtain drug history
Especially: Beta blockers, calcium channel blockers, digitalis, amiodarone, sotalol, other antiarrhythmic drugs. D/C unnecessary drugs.

Mobitz II or complete heart block with acute MI ?
No | Yes

Consider cardiac electrophysiologic testing

Symptoms due to bradycardia?
No | Yes

Minimal or no symptoms

Severe symptoms
Lightheadedness, reduced cardiac or urinary output, congestive heart failure

- First degree block
- Second degree Mobitz I block

Second degree Mobitz II or complete heart block. Resolved ?
Yes | No

IV atropine 0.5 - 1 mg IV
- Consider IV isoproterenol, epinephrine or dopamine
- Consider immediate transcutaneous pacing

persistent bradycardia

- Consider cardiac electrophysiologic testing
  Severe underlying conduction disorder?
No | Yes

- No therapy.
- Avoid drugs that can exacerbate AV conduction problems.

Review indications for permanent pacemaker (see *General Indications for Permanent Cardiac Pacemaker in Adults*)

IV Atropine: 0.5 - 1.0 mg IV push. Repeat every 3 - 5 min to a total of 0.04 mg / kg. More rapid dosing OK for severe bradycardia.
IV Isoproterenol: Infusion at 1 - 4 µg / min. May use doses as high as 10 µg / min for severe cases.
IV Epinephrine: 1 mg IV push. Repeat every 3 - 5 min. Higher doses of 3 - 5 mg IV push, up to a maximum bolus dose of 0.1 mg / kg.
CAUTION: Isoproterenol & epinephrine may exacerbate tachyarrhythmias, especially SVT, atrial fibrillation, and VT or VF.

Adult Advanced Cardiac Life Support. JAMA 1992; 268: 2199-2241.

2h: Bradycardia

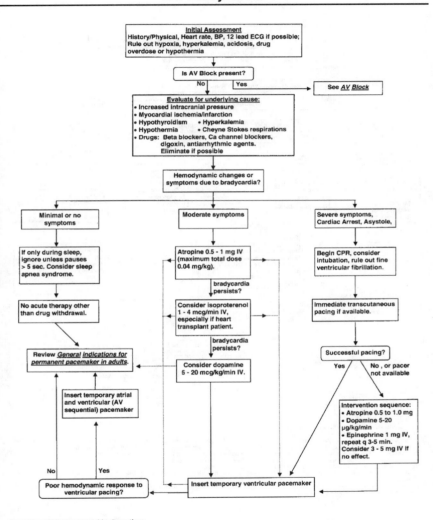

Initial Assessment
History/Physical, Heart rate, BP, 12 lead ECG if possible;
Rule out hypoxia, hyperkalemia, acidosis, drug
overdose or hypothermia

Is AV Block present?
No — Yes → See *AV Block*

Evaluate for underlying cause:
- Increased intracranial pressure
- Myocardial ischemia/infarction
- Hypothyroidism • Hyperkalemia
- Hypothermia • Cheyne Stokes respirations
- Drugs: Beta blockers, Ca channel blockers, digoxin, antiarrhythmic agents. Eliminate if possible

Hemodynamic changes or symptoms due to bradycardia?

Minimal or no symptoms

If only during sleep, ignore unless pauses > 5 sec. Consider sleep apnea syndrome.

No acute therapy other than drug withdrawal.

Review *General indications for permanent pacemaker in adults*.

Insert temporary atrial and ventricular (AV sequential) pacemaker

Moderate symptoms

Atropine 0.5 - 1 mg IV (maximum total dose 0.04 mg/kg).

bradycardia persists?

Consider isoproterenol 1 - 4 mcg/min IV, especially if heart transplant patient.

bradycardia persists?

Consider dopamine 5 - 20 mcg/kg/min IV.

Severe symptoms, Cardiac Arrest, Asystole,

Begin CPR, consider intubation, rule out fine ventricular fibrillation.

Immediate transcutaneous pacing if available.

Successful pacing?
Yes — No , or pacer not available

Intervention sequence:
- Atropine 0.5 to 1.0 mg
- Dopamine 5-20 µg/kg/min
- Epinephrine 1 mg IV, repeat q 3-5 min. Consider 3 - 5 mg IV if no effect.

No — Yes
Poor hemodynamic response to ventricular pacing?

Insert temporary ventricular pacemaker

Dotted lines indicate acceptable alternatives

Circulation, 2000; 102 (suppl I): I-140-157.

2i: Ventricular Arrhythmias

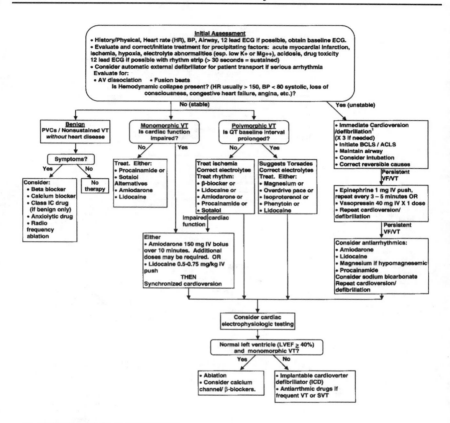

Initial Assessment
- History/Physical, Heart rate (HR), BP, Airway, 12 lead ECG if possible, obtain baseline ECG.
- Evaluate and correct/initiate treatment for precipitating factors: acute myocardial infarction, ischemia, hypoxia, electrolyte abnormalities (esp. low K+ or Mg++), acidosis, drug toxicity 12 lead ECG if possible with rhythm strip (> 30 seconds = sustained)
- Consider automatic external defibrillator for patient transport if serious arrhythmia
  Evaluate for:
  - AV dissociation   • Fusion beats
    Is Hemodynamic collapse present? (HR usually > 150, BP < 80 systolic, loss of consciousness, congestive heart failure, angina, etc.)?

No (stable) ———————————————— **Yes (unstable)**

Benign
PVCs / Nonsustained VT *without* heart disease

Symptoms?
Yes / No

Consider:
- Beta blocker
- Calcium blocker
- Class IC drug (if benign only)
- Anxiolytic drug
- Radio frequency ablation

No therapy

Monomorphic VT
Is cardiac function impaired?
No / Yes

Treat. Either:
- Procainamide or
- Sotalol
Alternatives
- Amiodarone
- Lidocaine

Impaired cardiac function

Either
- Amiodarone 150 mg IV bolus over 10 minutes. Additional doses may be required. OR
- Lidocaine 0.5-0.75 mg/kg IV push

THEN
Synchronized cardioversion

Polymorphic VT
Is QT baseline interval prolonged?
No / Yes

Treat ischemia
Correct electrolytes
Treat rhythm:
- β-blocker or
- Lidocaine or
- Amiodarone or
- Procainamide or
- Sotalol

Suggests Torsades
Correct electrolytes
Treat. Either:
- Magnesium or
- Overdrive pace or
- Isoproterenol or
- Phenytoin or
- Lidocaine

- Immediate Cardioversion /defibrillation[1] (X 3 if needed)
- Initiate BCLS / ACLS
- Maintain airway
- Consider intubation
- Correct reversible causes

Persistent VF/VT

- Epinephrine 1 mg IV push, repeat every 3 – 5 minutes OR
- Vasopressin 40 mg IV X 1 dose
- Repeat cardioversion/ defibrillation

Persistent VF/VT

Consider antiarrhythmics:
- Amiodarone
- Lidocaine
- Magnesium if hypomagnesemic
- Procainamide
Consider sodium bicarbonate
Repeat cardioversion/ defibrillation

Consider cardiac electrophysiologic testing

Normal left ventricle (LVEF ≥ 40%) and monomorphic VT?
Yes / No

- Ablation
- Consider calcium channel/ β-blockers.

- Implantable cardioverter defibrillator (ICD)
- Antiarrhythmic drugs if frequent VT or SVT

VF – ventricular fibrillation. VT – ventricular tachycardia.
IV epinephrine: 1 mg IV push. May repeat in 3 - 5 min. Maximum bolus is 0.1 mg/kg.
IV lidocaine: 1 - 1.5 mg/kg IV push. Repeat: 0.5 - 0.75 mg/kg IV push q 5 - 10 min to a maximum of 3 mg/kg. Start infusion at 2 - 4 mg/min.
IV procainamide: 17 mg/kg IV at 25 mg / min maximum loading rate. 1 - 4 mg/min maintenance infusion. May cause hypotension.
IV bretylium: 5 - 10 mg/kg IV over 8 - 10 min. Maximum bolus is 30 mg/kg over 24 hours. May cause hypotension.
IV amiodarone: 150 - 300 mg IV over 10 - 20 min; 1 mg/min IV for 6 hours; 0.5 mg/min IV maintenance.
Sodium bicarbonate: 1 mEq/kg IV. Additional doses as required for acidosis.
1. Cardioversion: Synchronize for organized VT at 25 - 360 Joules. Asynchronous for VF at 200 - 360 Joules. Use sedation (e.g. benzodiazepine) ± analgesic agent.

Circulation, 2000; 102 (suppl I): I-142-171.

2j: Antiarrhythmic Drugs

Class Ia

Drug	Dose IV	Dose PO	Therapeutic Level
Quinidine	6 - 10 mg/kg very slow IV infusion as loading dose (at least 1 hour). Not usually used as IV therapy.	200 - 600 mg q6 hours immediate release; 200 - 648 mg q8 – 12h SR.	3 - 6 mcg/ml
Procainamide	15 mg/kg IV at 25 mg/min loading dose, then 1 - 5 mg/min infusion.	250 - 750 mg q4 - 6 hours immediate release; 500 - 1250 mg q6 – 12h SR	Procainamide 5 - 12 mcg/ml, NAPA 5 - 12 mcg/ml
Disopyramide	N/A	100 - 200 mg q6 hours immediate release; 200 - 400 mg q12 hours SR	3 - 8 mcg/ml

Class Ib

Lidocaine	1 mg/kg loading dose, 0.5 mg/kg 5-10 min later, followed by 1 - 4 mg/min maintenance infusion.	N/A	2 - 5 mcg/ml
Mexiletine	N/A	150 - 400 mg q8 hours with food	0.5 - 2 mcg/ml
Tocainide	N/A	400 - 600 mg q8-12 hours.	4 - 10 mcg/ml

Class Ic

Propafenone	N/A	150 - 300 q8 hours.	N/A
Flecainide	N/A	50 - 200 q12 hours.	0.3 - 1.0 mcg/ml.
Moricizine	N/A	200 - 300 mg q8 hours	N/A

Class II

Propranolol	0.5 - 2.0 mg slow push q2 - 4 hours.	10 - 80 mg q6 hours immediate release; 40 - 160 mg q12h or qd SR	N/A
Esmolol	500 mcg/kg/min for 1 minute loading dose, 50 - 200 mcg/kg/min maintenance infusion.	N/A	N/A
Metoprolol	5.0 mg slow push, up to maximum of 15 mg.	25 - 200 mg q12 hours immediate release; 50 - 400 mg qd SR	N/A

Class III

Bretylium	5 - 10 mg/kg loading dose; 1 - 2 mg/min maintenance infusion.	N/A	N/A
Sotalol	N/A	80 - 240 mg q12 hours	N/A
Ibutilide	1 mg over 10 min, may repeat x1 after additional 10 min. Use less if weight less than 60 kg.	N/A	N/A
Amiodarone	150 mg over 10 min loading dose, followed by 1.0 mg/min for 6 hours then 0.5 mg/min.	800 - 1600 mg loading dose in divided doses for 5 to 14 days, then 600 - 800 mg daily for 2 to 6 weeks, then 200 - 400 mg daily.	Amiodarone 0.8 - 1.5 mcg/ml, Desethylamiodarone similar

Class IV

Verapamil	2.5 - 5 mg slow push.	40 - 120 mg q8 hours immediate release; 120 - 240 mg qd - q12h SR	N/A
Diltiazem	10 - 20 mg slow push loading dose, then 5 - 15 mg/min infusion.	30 - 120 mg q6 - 8 hours immediate release; 120 - 360 mg qd SR	N/A

Miscellaneous

Adenosine	6 - 18 mg rapid push	N/A	N/A
Digoxin	0.125 - 0.5 mg slow push, up to 0.75 - 1.25 mg / 24 hours	0.125 - 0.375 mg daily	0.5 - 2.0 ng/ml.
Digoxin Antibodies	40 mg (1 vial) for each 0.6 mg of total body store of digoxin. 240 mg typical for adult toxicity except for intentional overdose.	N/A	N/A

N/A: not available or not released in the United States as of this writing. SR – sustained release

2k: General Indications for Permanent Cardiac Pacemaker Implantation in Adults

Complete AV block	Markedly prolonged infra-His conduction (HV interval > 100 ms.)
Second degree AV block, Mobitz 2 or Mobitz I if block intra-His or infra-His.	Pacing induced infra-His block
Bilateral bundle branch block after myocardial infarct	Sinus node dysfunction with symptomatic bradycardia
Transient advanced AV block with bundle branch block after myocardial infarction	Sinus node dysfunction with heart rates < 40 bpm as a result of necessary drug therapy
Persistent advanced AV block after myocardial infarct	Recurrent syncope due to carotid sinus syndrome with pauses > 3 sec
Bifascicular block with intermittent complete heart block and symptomatic bradycardia	Bifascicular block with syncope, no other cause identified
Bifascicular block with Mobitz 2 2nd degree AV block	For control of SVT or ventricular tachycardias uncontrolled by other means
Congenital Long QT syndrome	Hypertrophic cardiomyopathy uncontrolled by drug therapy

Indications for Cardiac Electrophysiologic Testing

Class I (Indicated by general consensus)
- Symptomatic patients with SND in whom SND has not been clearly established as a cause of symptoms.
- Symptomatic patients with AVB in whom His-Purkinje block is suspected as a cause of AVB.
- Symptomatic patients with AVB or bundle branch block in whom VT is suspected as a cause of symptoms.
- Frequent or poorly tolerated SVT unresponsive to drug therapy, to guide medical treatment or perform catheter ablation.
- Patients with WPW referred for catheter ablation due to life threatening or incapacitating arrhythmias or drug intolerance.
- To guide catheter ablative or surgical techniques for SVT or VT and assess the efficacy of such procedures.
- Sustained or symptomatic wide QRS tachycardias to establish a diagnosis and guide therapy.
- Survivors of cardiac arrest due to tachyarrhythmia not associated with, or greater than 48 hours after, acute myocardial infarction (MI).
- Patients with unexplained syncope and known or suspected heart disease with possible brady- or tachyarrhythmias.
- Documented pulse rate inappropriately rapid (> 150 beats/min) with no ECG documentation of arrhythmia.

Class II (Discretionary)
- Symptomatic patients with SND to exclude other arrhythmias (e.g., VT), to assess anterograde & retrograde conduction and vulnerability to atrial tachyarrhythmias to determine appropriate pacing mode, and to assess response to drug therapy.
- Patients with second or third degree AVB to assess the level of block to guide therapy, and to exclude junctional extrasystoles as a cause of pseudo AVB.
- Symptomatic patients with bundle branch block to assess the level and severity of block to guide therapy.
- SVT patients to assess the effect of antiarrhythmic drug therapy on SN function or AV conduction.
- Patients with accessory pathways to determine the type, number, and characteristics of the bypass tracts and determine the response to drug therapy.
- Asymptomatic patients with WPW with a family history of sudden death; to guide participation in high risk occupations or activities; or in those having other cardiac surgery to consider surgical ablation of the accessory pathway.
- Risk stratification for pts with a reduced left ventricular ejection fraction, especially due to coronary artery disease, and frequent ventricular ectopy or nonsustained VT, especially with a positive signal averaged ECG, who have an increased risk for sudden death.
- To guide drug therapy in patients with inducible sustained or symptomatic VT.
- Patients with PVCs or nonsustained VT and unexplained syncope or presyncope.
- Patients with unexplained syncope without structural heart disease.
- Patients surviving a cardiac arrest due to bradyarrhythmia.
- Sporadic, significant palpitations that cannot be documented on long-term ECG or event records.
- Identification of proarrhythmic (arrhythmia exacerbating) effects in patients who experience symptoms or sustained VT or cardiac arrest while on antiarrhythmic medications.
- Evaluation of patients undergoing implantation of antiarrhythmic devices, including ICDs, plus re-evaluation when antiarrhythmic drug therapy is changed in such patients.
- Patients with congenital complete AVB and a wide QRS escape rhythm.

Class III (Not indicated)
- Patients with SND or AVB when symptoms are clearly related to the arrhythmia, or when clearly caused by drugs or reversible causes (e.g., inferior myocardial infarction).
- Asymptomatic patients with sinus bradyarrhythmias or sinus pauses during sleep.
- First degree AVB or asymptomatic Mobitz I second degree AVB with a narrow QRS complex.
- Asymptomatic patients with transient AVB associated with sinus slowing, consistent with a vagal mechanism.
- Asymptomatic patients with IVCD, bundle branch block, or bifascicular block.
- Asymptomatic patients with WPW syndrome.
- Patients with supraventricular tachycardia with no evidence of pre-excitation, with sufficient information from surface ECG or monitor to determine appropriate therapy, and who can be easily controlled with vagal maneuvers or medications.
- Patients with congenital long QT syndrome, or those with symptomatic acquired long QT syndrome related to an identifiable cause.
- Asymptomatic patients with PVCs or nonsustained VT with structurally normal hearts.
- Patients with a known cause of syncope.
- Patients with sustained VT or VF due to acute myocardial infarction or to reversible electrolyte / metabolic / toxic causes.

AVB= atrioventricular block	ICD= implantable cardioverter – defibrillator	IVCD= intraventricular conduction delay
PVC= premature ventricular complex	SND= sinus nodal dysfunction	SVT= supraventricular tachycardia
VF= ventricular fibrillation	VT= ventricular tachycardia	WPW= Wolff - Parkinson - White syndrome

Gregoratos G et al. ACC/AHA Guidelines for Implantation of Cardiac Pacemakers and Antiarrhythmia Devices: A report of the American College of Cardiology/American Heart Association Task Force on Practice Guidelines (Committee on Pacemaker Implantation). J Am Coll Cardiol 31: 1175-1209, 1998

Endocarditis prophylaxis recommended for:	Endocarditis prophylaxis not recommended for:
• *Prosthetic cardiac valves • *Prior episode of bacterial endocarditis • *Surgical systemic-pulmonary shunts/conduits • *Complex cyanotic congenital heart diseases • Other congenital heart diseases as noted on right • Rheumatic/other acquired valvular dysfunction • Hypertrophic cardiomyopathy • Mitral valve prolapse with mitral regurgitation and/or thickened leaflets (or if confirmation of MR/ thickening not available, with immediate need for the procedure) *high risk patients	• Isolated atrial secundum septal defect • >6 months after repair of ASD, VSD, PDA • Prior coronary artery bypass grafts • Mitral valve prolapse without mitral regurgitation • Cardiac pacemakers • Functional/innocent heart murmurs • Implantable defibrillators • Prior rheumatic fever or Kawasaki's disease without valvular dysfunction

Procedures for which antibiotic prophylaxis is recommended:	Procedures for which prophylaxis is not recommended:
• Dental procedures likely to cause bleeding and/or bacteremia: Professional cleaning, extractions, periodontal procedures, implants, root canal beyond apex, subgingival surgery, orthodontic bands, intraligamentary injections oral surgery involving teeth or gums • Endoscopic retrograde cholangiography with biliary obstruction • Tonsillectomy/adenoidectomy • Surgery involving GI, biliary, or respiratory tracts • Rigid bronchoscopy • Sclerotherapy of esophageal varices • Esophageal stricture dilatation • Incision and drainage of abscesses • Operations involving infected soft tissue • Cystoscopy, urethral dilatation, or prostatic surgery • The following GU procedures only if local infection is present: urethral catheterization, urinary tract surgery, vaginal delivery	• Dental procedures unlikely to cause bleeding: Restorative dentistry (fillings), orthodontic adjustments, local oral anesthetic injection (except intraligamentary), intracanal endodontic treatment, placement of rubber dams, post-op suture removal, oral impressions, fluoride treatments, oral X-rays, loss of primary teeth, placement of removable orthodontic or prosthodontic appliances • Tympanostomy tube insertion • Endotracheal intubation • Flexible bronchoscopy (with or without biopsy)[†] • Cardiac catheterization • GI endoscopy (with or without biopsy)[†] • Ceasarean section • Transesophageal echocardiography • Incision and biopsy of surgically scrubbed skin • Cardiac catheterization/angioplasty/pacemaker/ defibrillators or stent implantation • Circumcision • The following GU procedures in the absence of local infection: urethral catheterization, D & C, vaginal delivery[†], therapeutic abortion, sterilization procedures, vaginal hysterectomy[†] and IUD insertion/removal [†] optional in high risk patients

Current Recommendations for Endocarditis Prophylaxis

Indication	Regimen
Dental, oral, respiratory tract or esophageal procedures	• Amoxicillin 2.0 g po 1 hr pre-procedure OR If penicillin allergic (choose one regimen)**: • Clindamycin 600 mg po 1 hr pre-procedure OR • Azithromycin 500 mg po 1 hr pre-procedure OR • Clarithromycin 500 mg po 1 hr pre-procedure
Dental, oral, or respiratory tract or esophageal procedures; patients NPO	• Ampicillin 2.0 g 30' pre-procedure IV or IM If penicillin allergic: • Clindamycin 600 mg IV within 30 minutes pre-procedure
Genitourinary and non esophageal gastrointestinal procedures: High risk patients	• Ampicillin 2.0 g IV or IM plus gentamicin 1.5 mg/kg (max 120 mg) 30' pre-procedure, then either amoxicillin 1 g po 6 hrs later or ampicillin 1 g IV 6 h later If penicillin allergic: • Vancomycin 1.0g IV given over 1-2 h, plus gentamicin 1.5 mg/kg (max 120 mg), complete infusion within 30 minutes of starting the procedure
Genitourinary and non esophageal gastrointestinal procedures: Moderate risk patients	• Amoxicillin 2.0 g po 1 hr pre-procedure OR • Ampicillin 2.0 g 30' pre-procedure IV or IM If penicillin allergic: • Vancomycin 1.0g IV 1 hr pre-procedure given over 1 hr, complete within 30 minutes of starting the procedure

** Cephalosporin recommendations are not listed because they should not be used in patients with immediate-type hypersensitivity reactions to penicillins

Abbreviations: ASD - atrial septal defect. VSD - ventricular septal defect. PDA - patent ductus arteriosus. D & C - dilation and curettage. IUD - intrauterine device. AHA - American Heart Association.
Tables list those selected procedures and conditions listed in references but are not all-inclusive. Vancomycin and gentamicin should be adjusted for renal impairment

Dajani AS, et al. Prevention of bacterial endocarditis. Recommendations by the American Heart Association. JAMA 277: 1794-1801, 1997 and 264:2919, 1990
Simmons NA. Recommendations for endocarditis prophylaxis. J Antimicrob Chemother 31:437, 1993

2m: Therapy for Infectious Endocarditis

Empiric Therapy for Infective Endocarditis (cultures pending)

Clinical situation	Likely organisms	Antibiotic regimen
Native valve endocarditis	Viridans streptococci Staphylococcus aureus Enterococci	Vancomycin 1 gm IV q12h + Gentamicin 3 mg/kg/d
Early prosthetic valve endocarditis (<2 mos)	Staphylococcus epidermidis Staphylococcus aureus Enterobacteriaciae Diptheroids	Vancomycin 1 gm IV q12h + Gentamicin 3 mg/kg/d +/- Rifampin 600 mg p.o. qd
Late prosthetic valve endocarditis (> 2 mos)	Viridans streptococci Staphylococcus epidermidis Staphylococcus aureus Enterococci	Vancomycin 1 gm IV q12h + Gentamicin 3 mg/kg/d +/- Rifampin 600 mg p.o. qd

Indications for Surgery in Infective Endocarditis

Indications for urgent surgery	Relative indications for surgery
• Refractory heart failure • Persistent bacteremia • Fungal endocarditis • No effective antimicrobial agent available • Prosthetic valve obstruction • Unstable prosthesis	• Nonstreptococcal endocarditis • Relapse • Intracardiac extension of infection • 2 or more systemic emboli • Echocardiogram: -Vegetations -Mitral valve preclosure • Early prosthetic valve endocarditis • Periprosthetic valve leak

Specific Therapy for Native Valve Endocarditis

Organism	Antibiotic regimen	Duration	Comments
Viridans streptococci or Streptococcus bovis (MIC < 0.1 ug/ml Penicillin G)	Penicillin G 2-3 MU IV q4h OR Ceftriaxone 2 g IV qd OR Penicillin G 2-3 MU IV q4h + Gentamicin 3 mg/kg/d OR Vancomycin 1 gm IV q12h	4 weeks 4 weeks 2 weeks 2 weeks 4 weeks	2-week regimen only if no extra-cardiac foci of infection or intra-cardiac abscesses. Vancomycin used for patients allergic to β-lactam antibiotics.
Viridans streptococci or Streptococcus bovis (MIC > 0.1 and < 0.5 ug/ml Penicillin G)	Penicillin G 3 MU IV q4h + Gentamicin 3 mg/kg/d OR Vancomycin 1 gm IV q12h	4 weeks 2 weeks 4 weeks	Vancomycin used for patients allergic to β-lactam antibiotics.
Viridans streptococci (MIC > 0.5 ug/ml Penicillin G) Enterococci Nutritionally variant viridans streptococci	Penicillin G 3-5 MU IV q4h + Gentamicin 3 mg/kg/d OR Ampicillin 2 gm IV q4h + Gentamicin 3 mg/kg/d OR Vancomycin 1 gm IV q12h + Gentamicin 3 mg/kg/d	4-6 weeks 4-6 weeks 4-6 weeks 4-6 weeks 4-6 weeks 4-6 weeks	Treatment of enterococci dependent on susceptibilities. Vancomycin used for patients allergic to β-lactam antibiotics or for penicillin-resistant enterococci.
Methicillin-susceptible staphylococcus aureus	Nafcillin or oxacillin 2 gm IV q4h + Gentamicin 3 mg/kg/d (optional) OR Cefazolin 2 gm IV q8h + Gentamicin 3 mg/kg/d (optional) OR Vancomycin 1 gm IV q12h	4-6 weeks 3-5 days 4-6 weeks 3-5 days 4-6 weeks	Aminoglycosides expedite clearance of bacteremia but no proven benefit in clinical outcome. Vancomycin used for patients allergic to β-lactam antibiotics.
Methicillin-resistant staph aureus	Vancomycin 1 gm IV q12h	4-6 weeks	

Specific Therapy for Prosthetic Valve Endocarditis

Organism	Antibiotic regimen	Duration	Comments
Viridans streptococci or Streptococcus bovis (MIC < 0.1 ug/ml Penicillin G)	Penicillin G 3-5 MU IV q4h + Gentamicin 3 mg/kg/d OR Vancomycin 1 gm IV q12h + Gentamicin 3 mg/kg/d	4-6 weeks 2 weeks 4-6 weeks 2 weeks	Vancomycin for patients allergic to β-lactam antibiotics.
Viridans streptococci or Streptococcus bovis (MIC > 0.1 ug/ml Penicillin G) Enterococci Nutritionally variant viridans streptococci	Penicillin G 3-5 MU IV q4h + Gentamicin 3 mg/kg/d OR Ampicillin 2 gm IV q4h + Gentamicin 3 mg/kg/d	6-8 weeks 6-8 weeks 6-8 weeks 6-8 weeks	Vancomycin 1 gm IV q12h can be substituted for penicillin in patients allergic to β-lactam antibiotics or those with penicillin-resistant enterococci.
Methicillin-susceptible staphylococcus aureus	Nafcillin or oxacillin 2 gm IV q4h + Rifampin 600 mg p.o. qd + Gentamicin 3 mg/kg/d	6-8 weeks 6-8 weeks 2 weeks	Cefazolin 2 gm IV q8h substituted for nafcillin in patients with penicillin allergy. Vancomycin 1 gm IV q12h allergic to β-lactam antibiotics.
Methicillin-resistant staphylococcus aureus Coagulase-negative staphylococci	Vancomycin 1 gm IV q12h + Rifampin 600 mg p.o. qd + Gentamicin 3 mg/kg/d	6-8 weeks 6-8 weeks 2 weeks	Rifampin and gentamicin used in methicillin-resistant staphylococcus aureus infection only if organism susceptible.

Wilson WR, et.al. Antibiotic Treatment of Adults with Infective Endocarditis due to Streptococci, Enterococci, Staphylococci, and HACEK Microorganisms. JAMA 274:1706, 1995
Alsip SG, et. al. Indications for Cardiac Surgery in Patients with Active Infectious Endocarditis. Amer J Med 78:138, 1985

2n: Peripheral Arterial Disease

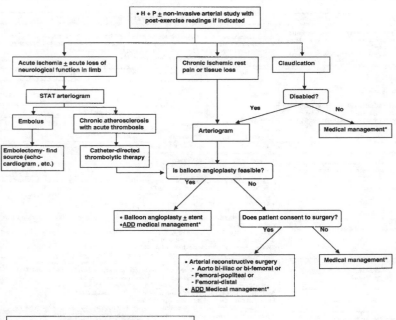

• H + P ± non-invasive arterial study with
post-exercise readings if indicated

Acute ischemia ± acute loss of
neurological function in limb

STAT arteriogram

Embolus

Chronic atherosclerosis
with acute thrombosis

Embolectomy- find
source (echo-
cardiogram , etc.)

Catheter-directed
thrombolytic therapy

Chronic ischemic rest
pain or tissue loss

Claudication

Disabled?

Yes   No

Arteriogram   Medical management*

Is balloon angioplasty feasible?

Yes   No

• Balloon angioplasty ± stent
•ADD medical management*

Does patient consent to surgery?

Yes   No

• Arterial reconstructive surgery
  - Aorto bi-iliac or bi-femoral or
  - Femoral-popliteal or
  - Femoral-distal
• ADD Medical management*

Medical management*

•MEDICAL MANAGEMENT
•Walking exercise program
•Prophylactic foot care
•Anti-platelet agent
  ‣ Enteric coated aspirin 81 or 325 mg/day or
  ‣ Clopidogrel 75 mg once/day
• ± Cilostazol (if no CHF) 50-100 mg bid ½ hour after meals
• Control risk factors (diabetes, blood pressure, weight, etc.)

Creager MA. Clinical assessment of the patient with claudication: the role of the vascular laboratory. Vasc Med. 1997;2(3):231-7.
Hiatt WR. Current and future drug therapies for claudication. Vasc Med. 1997;2(3):257-62.
DeWeese JA, et al. Practice guidelines: lower extremity revascularization. J Vasc Surg. 1993 Aug;18(2):280-94.
Palmaz JC, et al. Stenting of the iliac arteries with the Palmaz stent: experience from a multicenter trial. Cardiovasc Intervent Radiol. 1992 Sep-Oct;15(5):291-7.

2o: Antithrombotic Therapy: Common Indications and Recommended Therapy

Clinical disorder or indication	Recommended Therapy (alternative options)		
Stroke prevention after transient ischemic attack or stroke (see *Acute stroke* for acute treatment, and *Secondary prevention of ischemic stroke* for discussion of options)	Aspirin 75-1,300 mg/day Aspirin/extended release dipyridamole 200 mg – high risk for recurrent stroke Clopidogrel 75 mg qd (Ticlopidine 250 mg BID)- aspirin failure/contraindicated, or high risk (Aspirin plus clopidogrel 75 mg qd) – high risk for recurrent stroke Warfarin, INR 2-3: Aspirin failure or contraindication		
Asymptomatic carotid stenosis	Aspirin 325 mg/day (Aspirin 75-1,300 mg/day)		
	Age	**Risk factors**	**Recommendation**
Atrial fibrillation (AF) Risk factors: prior TIA, stroke, systemic embolism, hypertension, CHF, rheumatic mitral valve disease, prosthetic heart valve	< 65 years	Absent	Aspirin 325 mg qd
		Present	Warfarin, INR 2.0-3.0 (target 2.5)
	65-75 years	Absent	Aspirin or warfarin
		Present	Warfarin, INR 2.0-3.0 (target 2.5)
	> 75 years	All patients	Warfarin INR 2.0-3.0 (target 2.5)
Atrial fibrillation: Elective cardioversion	> 2 days AF: Warfarin, INR 2.0-3.0 X 3 weeks prior to cardioversion. Continue anticoagulation after cardioversion until in sinus rhythm for 4 weeks. < 2 days of SVT or AF: No therapy		
Stable angina / coronary artery disease	Aspirin 160-325 mg/day		
Unstable angina	ASA 160-325 mg/d or Clopidogrel 75 mg qd or Ticlopidine 250 mg bid, plus either heparin 75 U/kg bolus, then 1,250 U/h, adjust to APTT 1.5-2.0 X control, dalteparin120 IU/kg SC (max 10,000 IU) q12h, or enoxaparin 1 mg/kg SC q12h for 3-4 days or until syndrome resolves.		
Deep venous thrombosis	• Low molecular weight heparin (e.g. Enoxaparin 1 mg/kg SC q12h or 1.5 mg/kg q24h; or Tinzaparin 175 IU/kg SC q24h) • Heparin: 5-10,000 load, then 1,300 U/H, check and adjust Q6H until APTT 1.5-2.5 X control. Continue 4-7 days with warfarin, INR 2.0-3.0 OR • Warfarin: Start 5-10 mg with heparin or enoxaparin therapy, then adjust daily to INR 2.0-3.0 X 3 - 6 months, or long term if continued risk Thrombolytic Rx (when indicated): rtPA: 100 mg infused over 2 H[1] Restart heparin without a load once APTT or thrombin time < 1.5 X control		
Pulmonary embolism (See *Mangement of pulmonary embolism*)	• Heparin or low molecular weight heparin: dose as for deep venous thrombosis. • Warfarin: Start with heparin therapy at 5-10 mg, then adjust daily to INR 2.0-3.0 X 6 mos Thrombolytic Rx (when indicated): rtPA: 100 mg infused over 2 H[1] Restart heparin without a load once APTT or thrombin time < 1.5 X control		
Rheumatic mitral valve disease	Systemic embolism or atrial fibrillation: Warfarin, INR 2.0-3.0, target 2.5 Left atrial diameter > 5.5 cm: Warfarin, INR 2.0-3.0, target 2.5 Add aspirin (80-100 mg/d), clopidogrel 75 mg qd, or ticlopidine 250 bid if warfarin failure		
Mitral annular calcification	Systemic embolism hx or associated atrial fibrillation: Warfarin INR 2.0-3.0 Not recommended if no h/o embolism or atrial fibrillation		
Mitral valve prolapse	Not recommended if no h/o systemic embolism, TIAs or atrial fibrillation Unexplained TIAs: Aspirin 160-325 mg/d Systemic embolism, a fib, or recurrent TIAs despite ASA: Warfarin INR 2.0-3.0		
Patent foramen ovale (PFO) or Atrial septal defect	Asymptomatic: Not recommended Unexplained TIAs, venous thrombosis, pulmonary/systemic embolism: Warfarin INR 2.0-3.0 (unless venous interruption or closure of PFO is considered preferable)		
Bioprosthetic mitral valve/sinus rhythm	Mitral, sinus rhythm: Warfarin, INR 2.0-3.0 X 3 mos post op; Aspirin 162 mg/d long term Aortic, sinus rhythm: Warfarin; INR 2.0 – 3.0 X 3 mos optional; ASA 162 mg/d long term With a fib or systemic embolization: Warfarin INR 2.0 – 3.0 long term		
Prosthetic heart valves	Bileaflet aortic, normal L atrium, EF, and sinus rhythm: Warfarin, INR 2.0 – 3.0 (target 2.5) Tilting disk, bileaflet mitral valve, or bileaflet aortic with AF: Warfarin 2.5-3.5 (target 3.0) (Tilting disk, any bileaflet plus AF: Warfarin 2.0-3.0 (target 2.5) plus aspirin 80-100 mg/d) Caged ball or caged disk: Warfarin 2.5-3.5 (target 3.0) plus aspirin 80-100 mg/d Any valve plus additional risk factor: Warfarin 2.5-3.5 (target 3.0) plus aspirin 80-100 mg/d		
Myocardial infarction (see *Acute Myocardial infarction* for indications)	Heparin: load and maintenance as for deep venous thrombosis. rtPA: 15 mg IV bolus, then 0.75 mg/kg (but not > 50 mg) over 30 minutes, then 0.5 mg/kg (but not > 35 mg) over 60 minutes; OR APSAC 30 U IV over 5 minutes[1]		
Multiple Trauma	Enoxaparin 3,000 units bid; start 12-36 hours post injury		
Acute spinal injury	Enoxaparin 3,000 units bid		

1. Streptokinase and Urokinase are not available at publication date.
Note: Warfarin should not be during pregnancy. Heparin should be given during pregnancy when antithrombotic therapy is indicated.
Fifth ACCP consensus conference on antithrombotic therapy. Chest 114(suppl): 439S - 769S, 1998

3a: Management of Acute Pulmonary Thromboembolism

Determine clinical suspicion based on:
- History: Sudden onset dyspnea, syncope, substernal chest pain. If pleuritic pain, hemoptysis, likely infarction.
- Physical exam: Tachycardia, tachypnea. Massive PE: RV S3. Pleural rub suggests infarction.
- Lab: 1) ABG: ↓ PO2, ↓ PCO2, widened A-a gradient. 2) D-dimer by ELISA >500 ng/ml; if <500 ng/ml, PE unlikely.
- CXR: often normal or nonspecific; may see infiltrate and/or effusion with infarction.

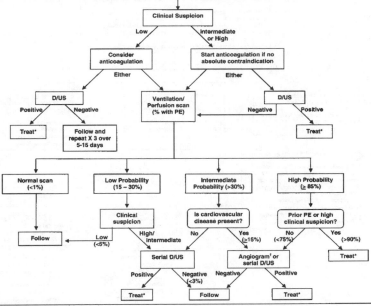

Indications for inferior vena cava filter:
- PE with contraindication to, or complication from, anticoagulation
- Massive PE in a patient in whom a subsequent PE might be fatal
- Consider in high risk patients with: chronic pulmonary hypertension, prior to pulmonary embolectomy, severe spinal, head, pelvic trauma, "free floating" thrombus
- Recurrent pulmonary embolism despite adequate anticoagulation
- Venogram-documented DVT with contraindication to heparin

D/US: Duplex ultrasound. PE: pulmonary embolism. PE likelihood is indicated in parenthesis (Kelly et al).
†Helical CT may be useful to detect central thromboembolism. Value is not established for peripheral emboli.
*Treat:
- If hemodynamically stable: Either (a) Low molecular weight heparin: Enoxaparin 1 mg/kg SC q12h or Tinzaparin 750 U/kg SC q 24h (both currently FDA approved for PE with DVT). Start warfarin within 24 h of dx and overlap with heparin or low molecular weight heparin for at least 5 days OR (b) Heparin 5,000 – 10,000U bolus then 1,300 U/h or 80U/kg bolus then 18 U/kg/h. ✓aPTT 6 hr after bolus or dosage change.
- If hemodynamically unstable ± RV hypokinesis on echocardiogram: Consider thrombolytic therapy if no contraindications: rTPA 100 mg continuous peripheral infusion over 2 h. No need to follow aPTT with infusion, but check at end and q4h prn until aPTT <80sec; then start heparin without bolus at 18 U/kg/h or 1,300 U/h.
- If anticoagulation contraindicated: place inferior vena cava filter

Hyers TM. Venous Thromboembolism: State of the Art. Am J Resp Crit Care Med 159: 1-14, 1999
Goldhaber SZ. Contemporary pulmonary embolism thrombolysis. Chest 107: 45S, 1995
Kelley MA et al. Diagnosing pulmonary embolism: New facts and strategies. Ann Intern Med 114: 300, 1991
Becker DM et al. Inferior vena cava filters: Indications, safety, effectiveness. Arch Int Med 152: 1985, 1992

3b: Acute Exacerbation of Asthma

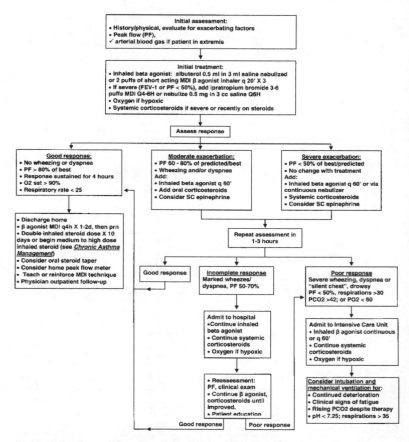

Initial assessment:
- History/physical, evaluate for exacerbating factors
- Peak flow (PF),
- ✓ arterial blood gas if patient in extremis

Initial treatment:
- Inhaled beta agonist: albuterol 0.5 ml in 3 ml saline nebulized or 2 puffs of short acting MDI β agonist inhaler q 20' X 3
- If severe (FEV-1 or PF < 50%), add ipratropium bromide 3-6 puffs MDI Q4-6H or nebulize 0.5 mg in 3 cc saline Q6H
- Oxygen if hypoxic
- Systemic corticosteroids if severe or recently on steroids

Assess response

Good response:
- No wheezing or dyspnea
- PF > 80% of best
- Response sustained for 4 hours
- O2 sat > 90%
- Respiratory rate < 25

Moderate exacerbation:
- PF 60 - 80% of predicted/best
- Wheezing and/or dyspnea
Add:
- Inhaled beta agonist q 60'
- Add oral corticosteroids
- Consider SC epinephrine

Severe exacerbation:
- PF < 50% of best/predicted
- No change with treatment
Add:
- Inhaled beta agonist q 60' or via continuous nebulizer
- Systemic corticosteroids
- Consider SC epinephrine

- Discharge home
- β agonist MDI q4h X 1-2d, then prn
- Double inhaled steroid dose X 10 days or begin medium to high dose inhaled steroid (see *Chronic Asthma Management*)
- Consider oral steroid taper
- Consider home peak flow meter
- Teach or reinforce MDI technique
- Physician outpatient follow-up

Repeat assessment in 1-3 hours

Good response

Incomplete response
Marked wheezes/ dyspnea, PF 50-70%

Poor response
Severe wheezing, dyspnea or "silent chest", drowsy
PF < 50%, respirations >30
PCO2 >42; or PO2 < 60

Admit to hospital
- Continue inhaled beta agonist
- Continue systemic corticosteroids
- Oxygen if hypoxic

Admit to Intensive Care Unit
- Inhaled β agonist continuous or q 60'
- Continue systemic corticosteroids
- Oxygen if hypoxic

- Reassessment:
PF, clinical exam
- Continue β agonist, corticosteroids until improved.
- Patient education

Consider intubation and mechanical ventilation for:
- Continued deterioration
- Clinical signs of fatigue
- Rising PCO2 despite therapy
- pH < 7.25; respirations > 35

Good response **Poor response**

- Corticosteroids: Recommended minimum dose - methylprednisolone 120-180 mg/day divided Q6-8H X 48 hours, then 50-80 mg/d until PF ≥ 70% of personal best or predicted
- Epinephrine dose: 0.3 mg of 1:1,000 dilution subcutaneously (SC) Q 20' X 3 doses
- Continuous β agonist: Withdraw 16 ml normal saline from 100ml bag; replace with 16 ml albuterol solution; run at 12.5 ml/hr into nebulizer ≈ 2 mg albuterol/hour
- Inhaled ipratropium: Ipratropium bromide 3-6 puffs MDI Q4-6H or nebulize 0.5 mg in 3 cc saline Q6H;

Guidelines for the diagnosis and management of asthma, NIH publication No. 97-4051, 1997
International consensus report on diagnosis and treatment of asthma; NIH Publication No. 92-3091, 1992
Manthous CA. Management of severe exacerbations of asthma. Am J Med 99:298; 1995

3c: Chronic Asthma Management

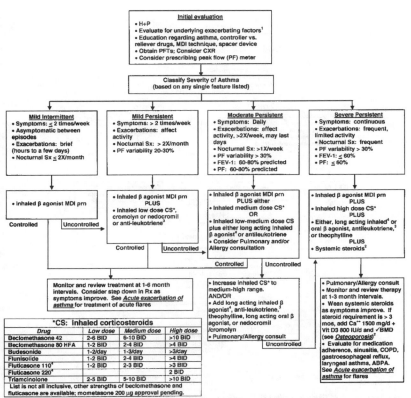

Initial evaluation
- H+P
- Evaluate for underlying exacerbating factors[1]
- Education regarding asthma, controller vs. reliever drugs, MDI technique, spacer device
- Obtain PFTs; Consider CXR
- Consider prescribing peak flow (PF) meter

Classify Severity of Asthma
(based on any single feature listed)

Mild Intermittent
- Symptoms: ≤ 2 times/week
- Asymptomatic between episodes
- Exacerbations: brief (hours to a few days)
- Nocturnal Sx ≤ 2X/month

Mild Persistent
- Symptoms: > 2 times/week
- Exacerbations: affect activity
- Nocturnal Sx: > 2X/month
- PF variability 20-30%

Moderate Persistent
- Symptoms: Daily
- Exacerbations: affect activity, >2X/week, may last days
- Nocturnal Sx: >1X/week
- PF variability > 30%
- FEV-1: 60-80% predicted
- PF: 60-80% predicted

Severe Persistent
- Symptoms: continuous
- Exacerbations: frequent, limited activity
- Nocturnal Sx: frequent
- PF variability > 30%
- FEV-1: ≤ 60%
- PF: ≤ 60%

- Inhaled β agonist MDI prn

Controlled | Uncontrolled

- Inhaled β agonist MDI prn PLUS
- Inhaled low dose CS*, cromolyn or nedocromil or anti-leukotriene[3]

Controlled | Uncontrolled

- Inhaled β agonist MDI prn PLUS either
- Inhaled medium dose CS* OR
- Inhaled low-medium dose CS plus either long acting inhaled β agonist[4] or antileukotriene
- Consider Pulmonary and/or Allergy consultation

Controlled | Uncontrolled

- Inhaled β agonist MDI prn PLUS
- Inhaled high dose CS* PLUS
- Either, long acting inhaled[4] or oral β agonist, antileukotriene,[3] or theophylline PLUS
- Systemic steroids[2]

Monitor and review treatment at 1-6 month intervals. Consider step down in Rx as symptoms improve. See *Acute exacerbation of asthma* for treatment of acute flares

- Increase inhaled CS* to medium-high range. AND/OR
- Add long acting inhaled β agonist[4], theophylline, long acting oral β agonist, or cromolyn
- Pulmonary/Allergy consult

Uncontrolled

- Pulmonary/Allergy consult
- Monitor and review therapy at 1-3 month intervals.
- Wean systemic steroids as symptoms improve. If steroid requirement is > 3 mos, add Ca⁺⁺ 1500 mg/d + Vit D3 800 IU/d and √BMD (see *Osteoporosis*)[5]
- Evaluate for medication adherence, sinusitis, COPD, gastroesophageal reflux, laryngeal asthma, ABPA. See *Acute exacerbation of asthma* for flares

*CS: Inhaled corticosteroids			
Drug	Low dose	Medium dose	High dose
Beclomethasone 42	2-6 BID	6-10 BID	>10 BID
Beclomethasone 80 HFA	1-2 BID	2-4 BID	>4 BID
Budesonide	1-2/day	1-3/day	>3/day
Flunisolide	1-2 BID	2-4 BID	>4 BID
Fluticasone 110⁴	1-2 BID	2-3 BID	>3 BID
Fluticasone 220⁴			2 BID
Triamcinolone	2-5 BID	5-10 BID	>10 BID

List is not all inclusive, other strengths of beclomethasone and fluticasone are available; mometasone 200 µg approval pending.

1. Exacerbating factors: β blockers, sinusitis, allergen exposure (e.g. cats, dogs, dust mite, cockroach, mold spores, etc.), gastro-esophageal reflux. Sinus CT, pH probe or trial of anti-reflux therapy, and/or skin or in-vitro testing to inhalant allergens may be helpful. Asthmatics sensitive to aspirin and NSAIDS should avoid their use. Exercise / cold air may precipitate symptoms in many patients.
2. Prednisone, methylprednisolone or prednisolone, 7.5-60 mg/d, use minimum effective dose (preferably alternate day therapy). Consider Calcium/Vitamin D3 on all patients (especially female) prescribed steroids. Consider Ophthalmology consult
3. Montelukast 10 mg qd, Zafirlukast 20 mg bid, Zileuton 600 mg qid
β -agonist: Albuterol, albuterol HFA, pirbuterol, or terbutaline MDI inhaler, 2 puffs, or albuterol rotocap 1-2 capsules or albuterol solution 1.25-5 mg in 2-3 ml saline. β agonists may be administered Q4-6H prn. Increasing use indicates "poor control".
4. Combination salmeterol/fluticasone dry powder inhaler is expected to be available shortly after publication
Long acting β agonist: Salmeterol 2 puffs MDI BID or 1 puff DPI BID; Fenoterol 1 puff BID, or oral sustained release albuterol 4-8 mg Q12H
Theophylline: 300-800 mg/day, use sustained release compound and aim for level of 8-12 mcg/ml
ABPA: Allergic Broncho-Pulmonary Aspergillosis. BMD: bone mineral densitometry

1998 Global Initiative for Asthma Report, World Asthma Meeting, 1998
Guidelines for the diagnosis and management of asthma, NIH publication No. 97-4051, 1997
International consensus report on diagnosis and treatment of asthma; NIH Publication No. 92-3091, 1992

3d: Management of Chronic Obstructive Pulmonary Disease

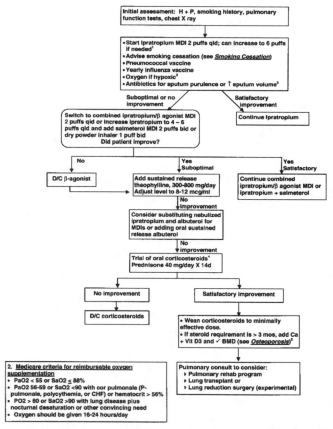

Initial assessment: H + P, smoking history, pulmonary function tests, chest X ray

- Start ipratropium MDI 2 puffs qid; can increase to 6 puffs if needed[1]
- Advise smoking cessation (see *Smoking Cessation*)
- Pneumococcal vaccine
- Yearly influenza vaccine
- Oxygen if hypoxic[2]
- Antibiotics for sputum purulence or ↑ sputum volume[3]

Suboptimal or no improvement

Satisfactory improvement

Switch to combined ipratropium/β agonist MDI 2 puffs qid or increase ipratropium to 4 – 6 puffs qid and add salmeterol MDI 2 puffs bid or dry powder inhaler 1 puff bid
Did patient improve?

Continue Ipratropium

No

D/C β-agonist

Yes Suboptimal

Add sustained release theophylline, 300-800 mg/day Adjust level to 8-12 mcg/ml

Yes Satisfactory

Continue combined ipratropium/β agonist MDI or ipratropium + salmeterol

No improvement

Consider substituting nebulized ipratropium and albuterol for MDIs or adding oral sustained release albuterol

No improvement

Trial of oral corticosteroids[4] Prednisone 40 mg/day X 14d

No improvement

D/C corticosteroids

Satisfactory improvement

- Wean corticosteroids to minimally effective dose.
- If steroid requirement is > 3 mos, add Ca + Vit D3 and ✓ BMD (see *Osteoporosis*)[5]

2. **Medicare criteria for reimbursable oxygen supplementation**
- PaO2 < 55 or SaO2 ≤ 88%
- PaO2 56-59 or SaO2 <90 with cor pulmonale (P-pulmonale, polycythemia, or CHF) or hematocrit > 56%
- PO2 > 60 or SaO2 >90 with lung disease plus nocturnal desaturation or other convincing need
- Oxygen should be given 16-24 hours/day

Pulmonary consult to consider:
▸ Pulmonary rehab program
▸ Lung transplant or
▸ Lung reduction surgery (experimental)

1. Alternative initial agents: a. Short acting inhaled β agonist (intermittant dyspnea) b. Combined ipratropium/ β-agonist c. Salmeterol
3. 7 days of broad spectrum po agent e.g.: doxycycline 100 mg bid, trimethoprim sulfasoxazole 1 DS BID, amoxicillin/clavulinic acid 500 mg bid, 2nd generation cephalosporin, clarithromycin 250-500 mg bid, or azithromycin 500 mg on day 1 then 250 mg qd X 4 days, oral quinolone.
4. Prior to oral steroid use, consider following therapies of unproven benefit in attempt to avoid the need for systemic steroid therapy:
(a) inhaled corticosteroids: evidence is controversial. (b) Montelukast, or zafirlukast (anecdotal evidence; studies ongoing).
5. Consider using in all patients (especially female) on steroids: Calcium 1500 mg/d. Vitamin D3 800 IU/d. BMD – bone mineral densitometry

ATS. Standards for the diagnosis and care of patients with chronic obstructive lung disease. Am J Crit Care Med 152:S77-S120, 1995
Ferguson GT, Cherniack RM. Management of chronic obstructive pulmonary disease. N Engl J Med 328: 1017, 1993
Mahler DA, Donohue JF, Barbee RA et al. Efficacy of salmeterol xinafoate in the treatment of COPD. Chest 115: 957-65, 1999
Barnes P. Chronic obstructive pulmonary disease. N Engl J Med. 2000 Jul 27;343(4):269-80.

3e: Chronic Obstructive Pulmonary Disease - Acute Respiratory Failure

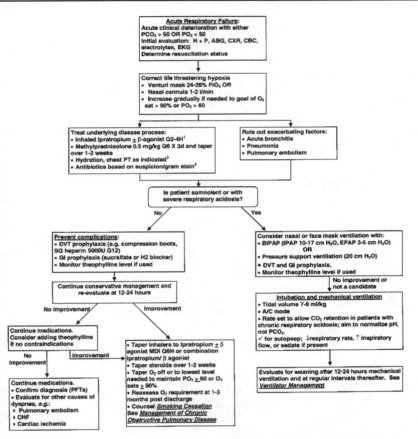

1. Ipratropium bromide MDI 2-6 puffs Q 4-6H or nebulize 0.5 mg solution; Albuterol MDI 2 puffs Q 2-4H or nebulize 0.5 ml of 0.5% solution
2. 7 days of broad spectrum po agent e.g. doxycycline 100 mg bid, trimethoprim sulfasoxazole 1 DS BID, amoxicillin/clavulinic acid 500 mg bid, 2nd generation cephalosporin, clarithromycin 250-500 mg bid, or azithromycin 250 mg, 2 on day 1 then 1 qd for 4 days, or quinolone (gatifloxacin 400 mg qd, levofloxacin or moxifloxacin 500 mg qd) (list not all-inclusive; cover *H. influenza*, *B. catarrhalis*, and *S. Pneumoniae*).
3. Chest PT may cause increased hypoxemia acutely.

Barnes P. Chronic obstructive pulmonary disease. N Engl J Med. 2000 Jul 27;343(4):269-80
Curtis JR, Hudson LD. Emergent assessment and management of acute respiratory failure in COPD. Clin Chest Med 15:481-497, 1994
Ferguson GT, Cherniack RM. Management of chronic obstructive pulmonary disease. N Engl J Med 328:1017-1022, 1993

3f: Interstitial Lung Disease: Diagnostic Evaluation

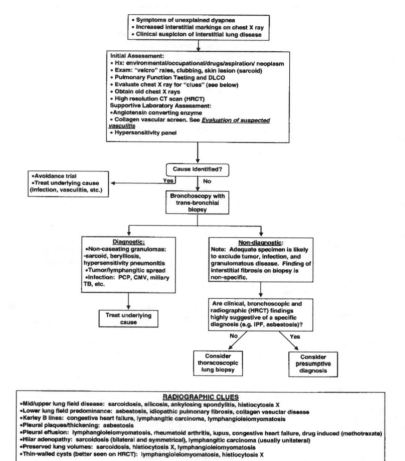

Symptoms of unexplained dyspnea
- Increased interstitial markings on chest X ray
- Clinical suspicion of interstitial lung disease

Initial Assessment:
- Hx: environmental/occupational/drugs/aspiration/ neoplasm
- Exam: "velcro" rales, clubbing, skin lesion (sarcoid)
- Pulmonary Function Testing and DLCO
- Evaluate chest X ray for "clues" (see below)
- Obtain old chest X rays
- High resolution CT scan (HRCT)

Supportive Laboratory Assessment:
- Angiotensin converting enzyme
- Collagen vascular screen. See *Evaluation of suspected vasculitis*
- Hypersensitivity panel

Cause identified? Yes / No

- Avoidance trial
- Treat underlying cause (infection, vasculitis, etc.)

Bronchoscopy with trans-bronchial biopsy

Diagnostic:
- Non-caseating granulomas:
  - sarcoid, berylliosis, hypersensitivity pneumonitis
- Tumor/lymphangitic spread
- Infection: PCP, CMV, miliary TB, etc.

Treat underlying cause

Non-diagnostic:
Note: Adequate specimen is likely to exclude tumor, infection, and granulomatous disease. Finding of interstitial fibrosis on biopsy is non-specific.

Are clinical, bronchoscopic and radiographic (HRCT) findings highly suggestive of a specific diagnosis (e.g. IPF, asbestosis)?   No / Yes

Consider thoracoscopic lung biopsy

Consider presumptive diagnosis

RADIOGRAPHIC CLUES
- Mid/upper lung field disease: sarcoidosis, silicosis, ankylosing spondylitis, histiocytosis X
- Lower lung field predominance: asbestosis, idiopathic pulmonary fibrosis, collagen vasuclar disease
- Kerley B lines: congestive heart failure, lymphangitic carcinoma, lymphangioleiomyomatosis
- Pleural plaques/thickening: asbestosis
- Pleural effusion: lymphangioleiomyomatosis, rheumatoid arthritis, lupus, congestive heart failure, drug induced (methotrexate)
- Hilar adenopathy: sarcoidosis (bilateral and symmetrical), lymphangitic carcinoma (usually unilateral)
- Preserved lung volumes: sarcoidosis, histiocytosis X, lymphangioleiomyomatosis
- Thin-walled cysts (better seen on HRCT): lymphangioleiomyomatosis, histiocytosis X

DLCO – diffusing capacity for carbon monoxide, PCP – pneumocystis pneumonia, CMV – cytomegalovirus, TB – tuberculosis, IPF – idiopathic pulmonary fibrosis, HRCT – high resolution CT scan

Schwarz M. Approach to the understanding, diagnosis and management of interstitial lung disease. In: *Interstitial Lung Disease*. Schwarz MI and King TE (eds). BC Decker. Hamilton. Ontario. 3rd edition. 1998.

3g: Treatment of Idiopathic Pulmonary Fibrosis

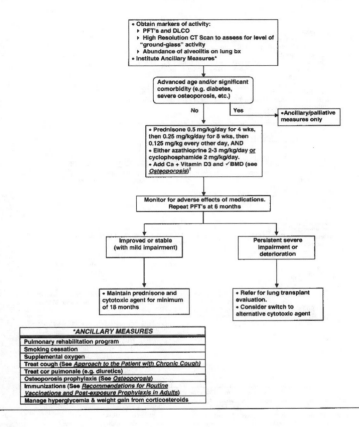

- Obtain markers of activity:
  - PFT's and DLCO
  - High Resolution CT Scan to assess for level of "ground-glass" activity
  - Abundance of alveolitis on lung bx
- Institute Ancillary Measures*

↓

Advanced age and/or significant comorbidity (e.g. diabetes, severe osteoporosis, etc.)

No → | Yes → •Ancillary/palliative measures only

↓

- Prednisone 0.5 mg/kg/day for 4 wks, then 0.25 mg/kg/day for 8 wks, then 0.125 mg/kg every other day, AND
- Either azathioprine 2-3 mg/kg/day or cyclophosphamide 2 mg/kg/day.
- Add Ca + Vitamin D3 and ✓BMD (see *Osteoporosis*)[†]

↓

Monitor for adverse effects of medications. Repeat PFT's at 6 months

↓

Improved or stable (with mild impairment) | Persistent severe impairment or deterioration

↓

- Maintain prednisone and cytotoxic agent for minimum of 18 months

- Refer for lung transplant evaluation.
- Consider switch to alternative cytotoxic agent

*ANCILLARY MEASURES
Pulmonary rehabilitation program
Smoking cessation
Supplemental oxygen
Treat cough (See *Approach to the Patient with Chronic Cough*)
Treat cor pulmonale (e.g. diuretics)
Osteoporosis prophylaxis (See *Osteoporosis*)
Immunizations (See *Recommendations for Routine Vaccinations and Post-exposure Prophylaxis in Adults*)
Manage hyperglycemia & weight gain from corticosteroids

† Ca++ 1500 mg/d + Vitamin D3 800 IU/d. BMD – bone mineral densitometry

Raghu G. Idiopathic pulmonary fibrosis: a rational clinical approach. Chest 92:148-154, 1987.
Raghu G, Depaso WJ, Cain K, et al. Azathioprine combined with prednisone in the treatment of idiopathic pulmonary fibrosis: a prospective double-blind, randomized, placebo-controlled clinical trial. Am Rev Respir Dis 144: 291-296, 1991.
Idiopathic Pulmonary Fibrosis: Diagnosis and Treatment. International Consensus Statement. Am J Respir Crit Care Med. 2000 Feb 1; 161 (2 Pt 1): 646-664.

3h: Treatment of Sarcoidosis

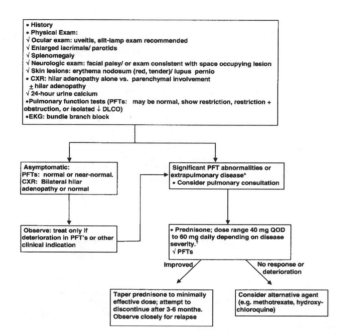

- History
- Physical Exam:
√ Ocular exam: uveitis, slit-lamp exam recommended
√ Enlarged lacrimals/ parotids
√ Splenomegaly
√ Neurologic exam: facial palsy/ or exam consistent with space occupying lesion
√ Skin lesions: erythema nodosum (red, tender)/ lupus pernio
- CXR: hilar adenopathy alone vs. parenchymal involvement
  ± hilar adenopathy
√ 24-hour urine calcium
- Pulmonary function tests (PFTs: may be normal, show restriction, restriction + obstruction, or isolated ↓ DLCO)
- EKG: bundle branch block

Asymptomatic:
PFTs: normal or near-normal.
CXR: Bilateral hilar adenopathy or normal

Significant PFT abnormalities or extrapulmonary disease*
- Consider pulmonary consultation

Observe: treat only if deterioration in PFT's or other clinical indication

- Prednisone; dose range 40 mg QOD to 60 mg daily depending on disease severity.[†]
√ PFTs

Improved

No response or deterioration

Taper prednisone to minimally effective dose; attempt to discontinue after 3-6 months. Observe closely for relapse

Consider alternative agent (e.g. methotrexate, hydroxy-chloroquine)

---

*Extrapulmonary Disease in Sarcoidosis:
- Includes central nervous system involvement, cardiac disease, liver involvement with marked derangements in liver function studies, posterior chamber uveitis, severe and disfiguring skin lesions, hypercalcemia refractory to dietary manipulation, or profound constitutional symptoms (weight loss, fevers, nightsweats, severe fatigue).
- Topical corticosteroids may be used for milder forms of cutaneous sarcoid and for anterior chamber uveitis.
- Nonsteroidal antiinflammatory agents may be used for painful erythema nodosum.

---

† If serum calcium not elevated, add calcium 1500 mg and Vitamin D3 800 IU/d supplementation and monitor serum calcium.
✓ bone densitometry. See *Osteoporosis*.

Kotloff RM and Rossman MD. Sarcoidosis. Immunol Allerg Clin North Amer 12:421-449, 1992.

3i: Pulmonary Hypertension

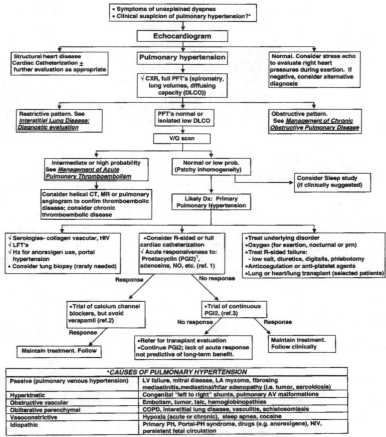

- Symptoms of unexplained dyspnea
- Clinical suspicion of pulmonary hypertension?*

Echocardiogram

Structural heart disease
Cardiac Catheterization ±
further evaluation as appropriate

Pulmonary hypertension

√ CXR, full PFT's (spirometry, lung volumes, diffusing capacity (DLCO))

Normal. Consider stress echo to evaluate right heart pressures during exertion. If negative, consider alternative diagnosis

Restrictive pattern. See: *Interstitial Lung Disease: Diagnostic evaluation*

PFT's normal or isolated low DLCO

Obstructive pattern. See *Management of Chronic Obstructive Pulmonary Disease*

V/Q scan

Intermediate or high probability
See *Management of Acute Pulmonary Thromboembolism*

Normal or low prob. (Patchy inhomogeneity)

Consider Sleep study (if clinically suggested)

Consider helical CT, MR or pulmonary angiogram to confim thromboembolic disease; consider chronic thromboembolic disease

Likely Dx: Primary Pulmonary Hypertension

√ Serologies- collagen vascular, HIV
√ LFT's
√ Hx for anorexigen use, portal hypertension
• Consider lung biopsy (rarely needed)

•Consider R-sided or full cardiac catheterization
√ Acute responsiveness to: Prostacyclin (PGI2)[1], adenosine, NO, etc. (ref. 1)

•Treat underlying disorder
•Oxygen (for exertion, nocturnal or prn)
•Treat R-sided failure:
  - low salt, diuretics, digitalis, phlebotomy
•Anticoagulation or anti-platelet agents
•Lung or heart/lung transplant (selected patients)

Response

No response

•Trial of calcium channel blockers, but avoid verapamil (ref.2)

•Trial of continuous PGI2, (ref.3)

Response

No response

Response

Maintain treatment. Follow

•Refer for transplant evaluation
•Continue PGI2; lack of acute response not predictive of long-term benefit.

Maintain treatment. Follow clinically

*CAUSES OF PULMONARY HYPERTENSION	
Passive (pulmonary venous hypertension)	LV failure, mitral disease, LA myxoma, fibrosing mediastinitis,mediastinal/hilar adenopathy (i.e. tumor, sarcoidosis)
Hyperkinetic	Congenital "left to right" shunts, pulmonary AV malformations
Obstructive vascular	Embolism, tumor, talc, hemoglobinopathies
Obliterative parenchymal	COPD, interstitial lung disease, vasculitis, schistosomiasis
Vasoconstrictive	Hypoxia (acute or chronic), sleep apnea, cocaine
Idiopathic	Primary PH, Portal-PH syndrome, drugs (e.g. anorexigens), HIV, persistent fetal circulation

PH – pulmonary hypertension. PFTs – pulmonary function testing. PGI2 – prostacyclin, NO – nitric oxide

1. Indications for PGI2 include PH from scleroderma, portal-PH and some congenital heart diseases with Eisenmenger's physiology

Palevsky HI. The treatment of Pulmonary Hypertension. *In:* Pulmonary Pharmacology and Therapeutics, AR Leff (ed), New York, McGraw Hill, 1996, pp. 1099-1109.

Rich S, Kaufmann E, Levy PA. The effect of high doses of calcium-channel blockers on survival in primary pulmonary hypertension. N Engl J Med 327:76-81, 1992.

Barst RJ, et al. A comparison of continuous intravenous epoprostenol (prostacyclin) with conventional therapy for primary pulmonary hypertension. N Engl J Med 334:296-301, 1996.

3j: Pleural Effusion

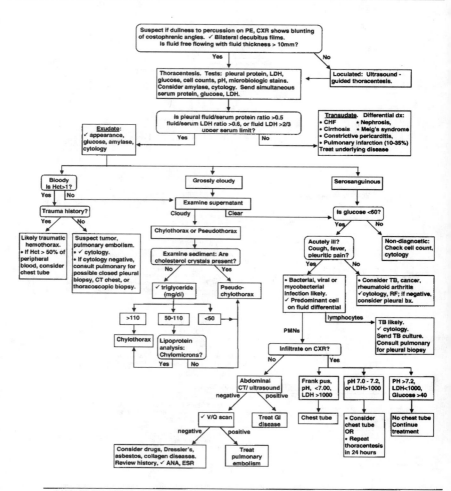

Suspect if dullness to percussion on PE, CXR shows blunting of costophrenic angles. ✓ Bilateral decubitus films. Is fluid free flowing with fluid thickness > 10mm?

Yes → Thoracentesis. Tests: pleural protein, LDH, glucose, cell counts, pH, microbiologic stains. Consider amylase, cytology. Send simultaneous serum protein, glucose, LDH.

No → Loculated: Ultrasound - guided thoracentesis.

Is pleural fluid/serum protein ratio >0.5 fluid/serum LDH ratio >0.6, or fluid LDH >2/3 upper serum limit?

Yes → Exudate:
✓ appearance, glucose, amylase, cytology

No → Transudate. Differential dx:
• CHF   • Nephrosis,
• Cirrhosis • Meig's syndrome
• Constrictive pericarditis,
• Pulmonary infarction (10-35%)
Treat underlying disease

Bloody
Is Hct>1?

Yes | No

Trauma history?
Yes | No

Likely traumatic hemothorax.
• If Hct > 50% of peripheral blood, consider chest tube

Suspect tumor, pulmonary embolism.
• ✓ cytology.
• If cytology negative, consult pulmonary for possible closed pleural biopsy, CT chest, or thoracoscopic biopsy.

Grossly cloudy

Examine supernatant
Cloudy | Clear

Chylothorax or Pseudothorax

Examine sediment: Are cholesterol crystals present?
No | Yes

✓ triglyceride (mg/dl) | Pseudo-chylothorax

>110 | 50-110 | <50

Chylothorax | Lipoprotein analysis: Chylomicrons?
Yes | No

Serosanguinous

Is glucose <60?
Yes | No

Acutely ill? Cough, fever, pleuritic pain?
Yes | No

Non-diagnostic: Check cell count, cytology

• Bacterial, viral or mycobacterial infection likely.
✓ Predominant cell on fluid differential

• Consider TB, cancer, rheumatoid arthritis
✓cytology, RF; if negative, consider pleural bx.

lymphocytes → TB likely.
✓ cytology.
Send TB culture.
Consult pulmonary for pleural biopsy

PMNs

Infiltrate on CXR?
No | Yes

Abdominal CT/ ultrasound
negative | positive

✓ V/Q scan | Treat GI disease
negative | positive

Consider drugs, Dressler's, asbestos, collagen diseases. Review history, ✓ ANA, ESR

Treat pulmonary embolism

Frank pus, pH, <7.00, LDH >1000

Chest tube

pH 7.0 - 7.2, or LDH>1000

• Consider chest tube
OR
• Repeat thoracentesis in 24 hours

PH >7.2, LDH<1000, Glucose >40

No chest tube
Continue treatment

1. Light, RW. Pleural Diseases 3rd edition. Baltimore, Williams and Wilkins, 1995.
2. Guidelines for Thoracentesis and Needle Biopsy of the Pleura. Am Rev Respir Dis. 140:257-258. 1989.

3k: Approach to the Patient with Chronic Cough

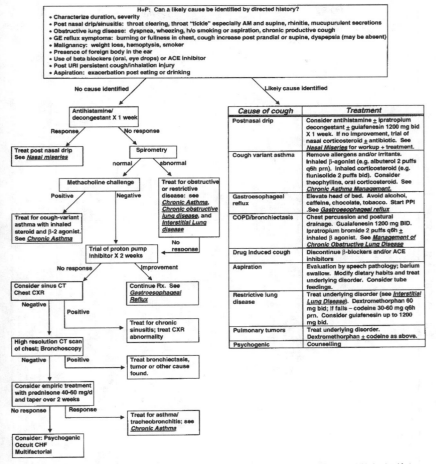

H+P: Can a likely cause be identified by directed history?

- Characterize duration, severity
- Post nasal drip/sinusitis: throat clearing, throat "tickle" especially AM and supine, rhinitis, mucupurulent secretions
- Obstructive lung disease: dyspnea, wheezing, h/o smoking or aspiration, chronic productive cough
- GE reflux symptoms: burning or fullness in chest, cough increase post prandial or supine, dyspepsia (may be absent)
- Malignancy: weight loss, hemoptysis, smoker
- Presence of foreign body in the ear
- Use of beta blockers (oral, eye drops) or ACE inhibitor
- Post URI persistent cough/inhalation injury
- Aspiration: exacerbation post eating or drinking

No cause identified → Likely cause identified

No cause identified branch:

Antihistamine/decongestant X 1 week

- Response → Treat post nasal drip. See *Nasal miseries*
- No response → Spirometry
  - normal → Methacholine challenge
    - Positive → Treat for cough-variant asthma with inhaled steroid and β-2 agonist. See *Chronic Asthma*
    - Negative → Trial of proton pump inhibitor X 2 weeks
      - No response → Consider sinus CT Chest CXR
        - Negative → High resolution CT scan of chest; Bronchoscopy
          - Negative → Consider empiric treatment with prednisone 40-60 mg/d and taper over 2 weeks
            - No response → Consider: Psychogenic, Occult CHF, Multifactorial
            - Response → Treat for asthma/tracheobronchitis; see *Chronic Asthma*
          - Positive → Treat bronchiectasis, tumor or other cause found.
        - Positive → Treat for chronic sinusitis; treat CXR abnormality
      - Improvement → Continue Rx. See *Gastroesophageal Reflux*
  - abnormal → Treat for obstructive or restrictive disease: see *Chronic Asthma*, *Chronic obstructive lung disease*, and *Interstitial Lung disease*

Likely cause identified branch:

Cause of cough	Treatment
Postnasal drip	Consider antihistamine ± ipratropium decongestant ± guiafenesin 1200 mg bid X 1 week. If no improvement, trial of nasal corticosteroid ± antibiotic. See *Nasal Miseries* for workup + treatment.
Cough variant asthma	Remove allergens and/or irritants. Inhaled β-agonist (e.g. albuterol 2 puffs q6h prn). Inhaled corticosteroid (e.g. flunisolide 2 puffs bid). Consider theophylline, oral corticosteroid. See *Chronic Asthma Management*.
Gastroesophageal reflux	Elevate head of bed. Avoid alcohol, caffeine, chocolate, tobacco. Start PPI. See *Gastroesophageal reflux*.
COPD/bronchiectasis	Chest percussion and postural drainage. Guaifenesin 1200 mg BID. Ipratropium bromide 2 puffs q6h ± inhaled β agonist. See *Management of Chronic Obstructive Lung Disease*
Drug induced cough	Discontinue β-blockers and/or ACE inhibitors
Aspiration	Evaluation by speech pathology; barium swallow. Modify dietary habits and treat underlying disorder. Consider tube feedings.
Restrictive lung disease	Treat underlying disorder (see *Interstitial Lung Disease*). Dextromethorphan 60 mg bid; if fails – codeine 30-60 mg q6h prn. Consider guiafenesin up to 1200 mg bid.
Pulmonary tumors	Treat underlying disorder. Dextromethorphan ± codeine as above.
Psychogenic	Counseling

Proton pump inhibitors. Omeprazole 20 mg or Lansoprazole 30 mg bid, or Rabeprazole 20 mg or Pantoprazole 40 mg qAM before breakfast

Smyrnios N, Irwin R, Curley F, French C. From a prospective study of chronic cough: Diagnostic and therapeutic aspects in older adults. Arch Int Med 158; 1222-1228, 1998.
Patrick H, Patrick F. Chronic cough. Med Clin North Amer 79:361-372, 1995
Pratter MR. Bartter. T. Akers S. et al. An algorithmic approach to chronic cough. Ann Intern Med 119:977-983. 1993.

3I: Solitary Pulmonary Nodule

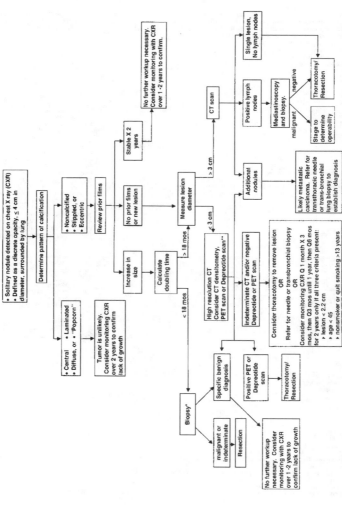

* Controversial. Some authors suggest fiberoptic bronchoscopy (for central lesions≥4 cm) or transthoracic needle biopsy (for peripheral lesions or if bronchoscopy is negative). Others suggest proceeding directly to resection, especially if clinical suspicion for malignancy is high. Isolated lesions with rapid doubling times (<7-21 days) are less likely to be malignant.

Midthun DE. Solitary Pulmonary nodule. www.chestnet.org/lesson18.html. 1997
Midthun DE, Swensen SJ, Jett FR. Approach to the Solitary Pulmonary Nodule. Mayo Clin Proc 68:378-385. 1993
Lillington GA. Management of Solitary Pulmonary Nodules. Dis Mon 37: 276-310, 1991
** Blum et al. A multicenter trial with a somatostatin analog 99mTC Depreotide in the evaluation of solitary pulmonary nodules. Chest 117: 1232-1238, 2000

3m: Workup and Treatment of Persistent and Intractable Hiccups

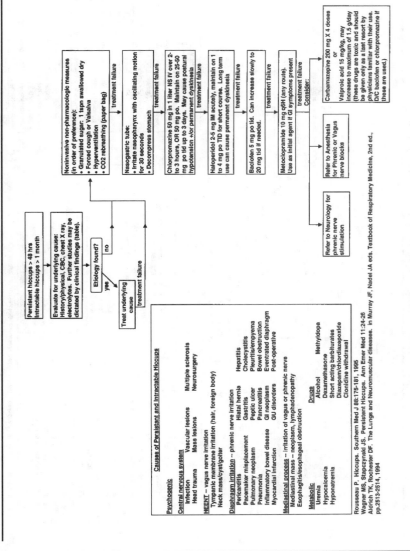

Persistent hiccups > 48 hrs
Intractable hiccups > 1 month

Evaluate for underlying cause:
History/physical, CBC, chest X ray, electrolytes. Further studies may be dictated by clinical findings (table).

Etiology found?

yes → Treat underlying cause
treatment failure

no

Noninvasive non-pharmacologic measures (in order of preference):
- Granulated sugar: 1 tspn swallowed dry
- Forced cough or Valsalva
- Hyperventilation
- CO2 rebreathing (paper bag)

treatment failure

Nasogastric tube:
- Irritate nasopharynx with oscillating motion for 30 seconds
- Decompress stomach

treatment failure

Chlorpromazine 50 mg in 1 liter NS IV over 2-to 3 hours, OR 50 mg po. Maintain on 25-50 mg po tid up to 3 days. May cause postural hypotension +/or permanent dyskinesia

treatment failure

Haloperidol 2-5 mg IM acutely, maintain on 1 to 4 mg po TID for short course. Long term use can cause permanent dyskinesia

treatment failure

Baclofen 5 mg po tid. Can increase slowly to 20 mg tid if needed.

treatment failure

Metoclopramide 10 mg q6H (any route).
Use as initial agent if GI symptoms present

treatment failure

Consider:

Carbamazepine 200 mg X 4 doses
or
Valproic acid 15 mg/Kg, may increase to maximum of 1.5 g/day (these drugs are toxic and should be given only as a last resort by physicians familiar with their use. D/C baclofen or chlorpromazine if these are used.)

Refer to Neurology for phrenic nerve stimulation

Refer to Anesthesia for Phrenic or Vagus nerve blocks

Causes of Persistent and Intractable Hiccups

Psychogenic

Central nervous system
Infection   Vascular lesions   Multiple sclerosis
Head trauma   Mass lesions   Neurosurgery

HEENT – vagus nerve irritation
Tympanic membrane irritation (hair, foreign body)
Neck mass/cyst/goiter

Diaphragm irritation – phrenic nerve irritation
Pericarditis   Hiatal hernia   Hepatitis
Pacemaker misplacement Gastritis   Cholecystitis
Pulmonary neoplasm   Peptic ulcer   Pleuritis/empyema
Pneumonia   Pancreatitis   Bowel obstruction
Inflammatory bowel disease GI neoplasm   Eventrated diaphragm
Myocardial Infarction   GU disorders   Post-operative

Mediastinal process – irritation of vagus or phrenic nerve
Mediastinal mass – neoplasm, lymphadenopathy
Esophagitis/esophageal obstruction

Metabolic
Uremia   Alcohol   Methyldopa
Hypocalcemia   Dexamethasone   Short acting barbiturates
Hyponatremia   Diazepam/chlordiazepoxide   Clonidine withdrawal

Drugs

Rousseau P. Hiccups. Southern Med J 88:175-181, 1995
Wagner MS, Stapczynski JS. Persistent Hiccups. Ann Emer Med 11:24-26
Aldrich TK, Rochester DF. The Lungs and Neuromuscular diseases. in Murray JF, Nadel JA eds. Textbook of Respiratory Medicine, 2nd ed., pp.2513-2514, 1994

3n: Evaluation and Management of Hemoptysis

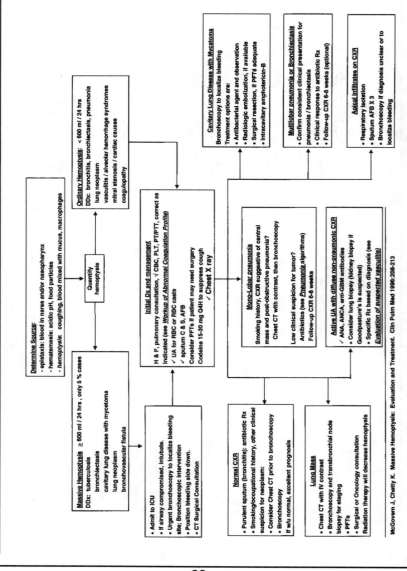

Determine Source:
- epistaxis: blood in nares and/or nasopharynx
- hematemesis: acidic pH, food particles
- *hemoptysis*: coughing, blood mixed with mucus, macrophages

Massive Hemoptysis: ≥ 600 ml / 24 hrs, only 5 % cases

DDx: tuberculosis
bronchiectasis
cavitary lung disease with mycetoma
lung neoplasm
bronchovascular fistula

Ordinary Hemoptysis: < 600 ml / 24 hrs
DDx: bronchitis, bronchiectasis, pneumonia
lung neoplasm
vasculitis / alveolar hemorrhage syndromes
mitral stenosis / cardiac causes
coagulopathy

Quantify hemoptysis

Initial Dx and management
H & P, pulmonary consultation, √ CBC, PLT, PT/PTT, correct as
indicated (see *Workup of Abnormal Coagulation Profile*)
√ UA for RBC or RBC casts
√ sputum C & S, AFB
Consider PFTs if patient may need surgery
Codeine 15-30 mg Q4H to suppress cough
√ Chest X ray

- Admit to ICU
- If airway compromised, intubate.
- Urgent bronchoscopy to localize bleeding
  site; Bronchoscopic intervention
- Position bleeding side down.
- CT Surgical Consultation

Cavitary Lung Disease with Mycetoma
Bronchoscopy to localize bleeding
Treatment options are:
- Antibacterial agent and observation
- Radiologic embolization, if available
- Surgical resection, if PFTs adequate
- Intracavitary amphotericin-B

Multilobar pneumonia or Bronchiectasis
- Confirm consistent clinical presentation for
  pneumonia / bronchiectasis
- Clinical response to antibiotic Rx
- Follow-up CXR 6-8 weeks (optional)

Apical Infiltrates on CXR
- Respiratory isolation
- Sputum AFB X 3
- Bronchoscopy if diagnosis unclear or to
  localize bleeding

Mono-Lobar pneumonia
Smoking history, CXR suggestive of central
mass and post-obstructive pneumonia?
Chest CT with contrast, then bronchoscopy

Low clinical suspicion for tumor?
Antibiotics (see *Pneumonia* algorithms)
Follow-up CXR 6-8 weeks

Active UA with diffuse non-pneumonic CXR
√ ANA, ANCA, anti-GBM antibodies
- Consider lung biopsy (kidney biopsy if
  Goodpasture's is suspected)
- Specific Rx based on diagnosis (see
  Evaluation of suspected vasculitis)

Normal CXR
- Purulent sputum (bronchitis): antibiotic Rx
- Smoking/occupational history, other clinical
  suspicion for neoplasm:
- Consider Chest CT prior to bronchoscopy
- Bronchoscopy
If w/u normal, excellent prognosis

Lung Mass
- Chest CT with IV contrast
- Bronchoscopy and transbronchial node
  biopsy for staging
- PFTs
- Surgical or Oncology consultation
Radiation therapy will decrease hemoptysis

McGovern J, Chetty K. Massive Hemoptysis: Evaluation and Treatment. Clin Pulm Med 1996:206-213

3o: Management of Community Acquired Pneumonia

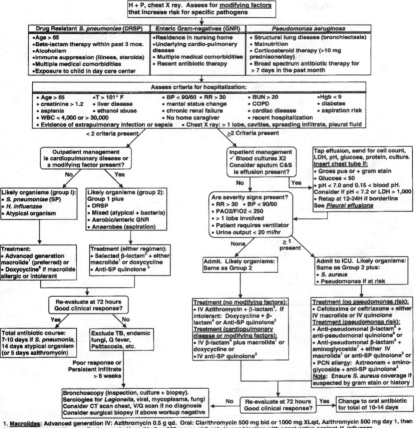

H + P, chest X ray. Assess for modifying factors that increase risk for specific pathogens

Drug Resistant S. pneumoniae (DRSP)	Enteric Gram-negatives (GNR)	Pseudomonas aeruginosa
• Age > 65 • Beta-lactam therapy within past 3 mos. • Alcoholism • Immune suppression (illness, steroids) • Multiple medical comorbidities • Exposure to child in day care center	• Residence in nursing home • Underlying cardio-pulmonary disease • Multiple medical comorbidities • Recent antibiotic therapy	• Structural lung disease (bronchiectasis) • Malnutrition • Corticosteroid therapy (>10 mg prednisone/day) • Broad spectrum antibiotic therapy for > 7 days in the past month

Assess criteria for hospitalization:

• Age > 65	• T > 101° F	• BP < 90/60	• RR > 30	• BUN > 20	• Hgb < 9
• creatinine > 1.2	• liver disease	• mental status change	• COPD	• cardiac disease	• diabetes
• asplenia	• ethanol abuse	• chronic renal failure		• recent hospitalization	• aspiration risk
• WBC < 4,000 or > 30,000		• No home caregiver			

• Evidence of extrapulmonary infection or sepsis • Chest X ray: > 1 lobe, cavities, spreading infiltrate, pleural fluid

< 2 criteria present

Outpatient management
Is cardiopulmonary disease or
a modifying factor present?

No → Likely organisms (group I):
• S. pneumoniae (SP)
• H. influenzae
• Atypical organism

Treatment:
• Advanced generation macrolide[1] (preferred) or
• Doxycycline[6] if macrolide allergic or intolerant

Yes → Likely organisms (group 2):
Group 1 plus
• DRSP
• Mixed (atypical + bacteria)
• Aerobic/enteric GNR
• Anaerobes (aspiration)

Treatment (either regimen):
• Selected β-lactam[4] + either macrolide[1] or doxycycline
• Anti-SP quinolone[3]

Re-evaluate at 72 hours
Good clinical response?

Yes → Total antibiotic course:
7-10 days if S. pneumonia,
14 days atypical organism
(or 5 days azithromycin)

No → Exclude TB, endemic fungi, Q fever, Psittacosis, etc.

Poor response or
Persistent infiltrate
> 6 weeks

≥2 Criteria present

Inpatient management
✓ Blood cultures X2
Consider sputum C&S
Is effusion present?

Yes → Tap effusion, send for cell count, LDH, pH, glucose, protein, culture.
Insert chest tube if:
• Gross pus or + gram stain
• Glucose < 50
• pH < 7.0 and 0.15 < blood pH.
Consider if pH < 7.2 or LDH > 1,000
• Retap at 12-24H if borderline
See Pleural effusions

No → Are severity signs present?
• RR > 30 • BP < 90/60
• PAO2/FIO2 < 250
• > 1 lobe involved
• Patient requires ventilator
• Urine output < 20 ml/hr

None → Admit. Likely organisms:
Same as Group 2

Treatment (no modifying factors):
• IV Azithromycin + β-lactam[4]. If intolerant: Doxycycline + β-lactam[4] or Anti-SP quinolone[3]
Treatment (cardiopulmonary disease or modifying factors):
• IV β-lactam[4] plus macrolide[1] or doxycycline or
• IV anti-SP quinolone[3]

≥ 1 present → Admit to ICU. Likely organisms:
Same as Group 2 plus:
• S. aureus
• Pseudomonas if at risk

Treatment (no pseudomonas risk):
• Cefotaxime or ceftriaxone + either IV macrolide or IV quinolone
Treatment (pseudomonas risk):
• Anti-pseudomonal β-lactam[5] + anti-pseudomonal quinolone[6] or
• Anti-pseudomonal β-lactam[5] + aminoglycoside[7] + either IV macrolide[1] or anti-SP quinolone[3] or
• PCN allergy: Aztreonam + amino-glycoside + anti-SP quinolone[3]
Note: Ensure S. aureus coverage if suspected by gram stain or history

Re-evaluate at 72 hours
Good clinical response?

No → Bronchoscopy (inspection, culture + biopsy).
Serologies for Legionella, viral, mycoplasma, fungi
Consider CT scan chest, V/Q scan if no diagnosis
Consider surgical biopsy if above workup negative

Yes → Change to oral antibiotic for total of 10-14 days

1. **Macrolides:** Advanced generation IV: Azithromycin 0.5 g qd. Oral: Clarithromycin 500 mg bid or 1000 mg XLqd, Azithromycin 500 mg day 1, then 250 mg qd X 4 days. May use Erythromycin (1 gm IV q6 or 500 mg po qid) only in combination with agent active against H. influenza.
2. **Selected β-lactams:** Amoxicillin 1 g po q8h (use with advanced macrolide), Amoxicillin/clavulanate 875 mg bid, Cefpodoxime 200 mg po q12h, cefuroxime 500 mg po q12h, or Ceftriaxone 1 gram IM or IV followed by po cefpodoxime.
3. **Anti-SP quinolones:** Gatifloxacin 400 mg qd, Levofloxacin 500 mg qd, Moxifloxacin 400 mg qd.
4. **IV β lactams:** Cefotaxime 2 g q4-8h, Ceftriaxone 1-2 g qd , Ampicillin/sulbactam 1.5 – 3.0 g q6h, Ampicillin 2g q6h (use with advanced macrolide)
5. **Antipseudomonal β lactams:** Cefepime 1.0-2.0 g q12h, Piperacillin/tazobactam 4.5g q6h, Ticarcillin/clavulanate 3.1 g q4-6h, Imipenem 0.5g Q6h, Meropenem 1g q12h
6. Ciprofloxacin 400mg IV q12h. Anti-SP quinolones may be effective against Pseudomonas but are not FDA approved for this indication.
7. **Other drugs.** Gentamicin or Tobramycin 3-5 mg/kg/d as single daily dose or divided into 2 or 3 doses. Amikacin 7.5mg/kg q12, not to exceed 1.5g/day. Adjust aminoglycosides to level and renal function. Doxycycline 100 mg bid. Aztreonam 2g IV q6h.

ATS Statement. Guidelines for the initial management of adults with community acquired pneumonia. Am J Resp Crit Care Med 2001 (pending)

3p: Nosocomial Pneumonia

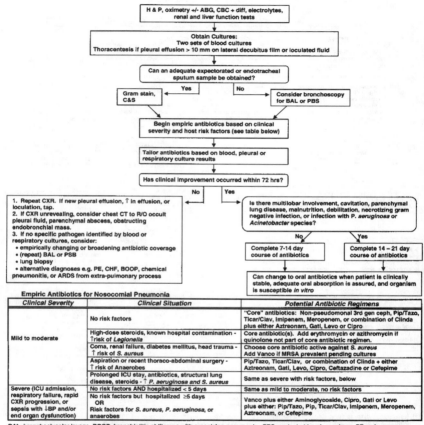

H & P, oximetry +/- ABG, CBC + diff, electrolytes, renal and liver function tests

↓

Obtain Cultures:
Two sets of blood cultures
Thoracentesis if pleural effusion > 10 mm on lateral decubitus film or loculated fluid

↓

Can an adequate expectorated or endotracheal sputum sample be obtained?

Yes → Gram stain, C&S

No → Consider bronchoscopy for BAL or PBS

↓

Begin empiric antibiotics based on clinical severity and host risk factors (see table below)

↓

Tailor antibiotics based on blood, pleural or respiratory culture results

↓

Has clinical improvement occurred within 72 hrs?

No:
1. Repeat CXR. If new pleural effusion, ↑ in effusion, or loculation, tap.
2. If CXR unrevealing, consider chest CT to R/O occult pleural fluid, parenchymal abscess, obstructing endobronchial mass.
3. If no specific pathogen identified by blood or respiratory cultures, consider:
   - empirically changing or broadening antibiotic coverage
   - (repeat) BAL or PSB
   - lung biopsy
   - alternative diagnoses e.g. PE, CHF, BOOP, chemical pneumonitis, or ARDS from extra-pulmonary process

Yes:
Is there multilobar involvement, cavitation, parenchymal lung disease, malnutrition, debilitation, necrotizing gram negative infection, or infection with P. aeruginosa or Acinetobacter species?

No → Complete 7-14 day course of antibiotics

Yes → Complete 14 – 21 day course of antibiotics

↓

Can change to oral antibiotics when patient is clinically stable, adequate oral absorption is assured, and organism is susceptible in vitro

Empiric Antibiotics for Nosocomial Pneumonia

Clinical Severity	Clinical Situation	Potential Antibiotic Regimens
Mild to moderate	No risk factors	"Core" antibiotics: Non-pseudomonal 3rd gen ceph, Pip/Tazo, Ticar/Clav, Imipenem, Meropenem, or combination of Clinda plus either Aztreonam, Gati, Levo or Cipro
	High-dose steroids, known hospital contamination - ↑risk of Legionella	Core antibiotic(s). Add erythromycin or azithromycin if quinolone not part of core antibiotic regimen.
	Coma, renal failure, diabetes mellitus, head trauma - ↑ risk of S. aureus	Choose core antibiotic active against S. aureus. Add Vanco if MRSA prevalent pending cultures
	Aspiration or recent thoraco-abdominal surgery - ↑ risk of Anaerobes	Pip/Tazo, Ticar/Clav, or combination of Clinda + either Aztreonam, Gati, Levo, Cipro, Ceftazadine or Cefepime
	Prolonged ICU stay, antibiotics, structural lung disease, steroids - ↑ P. aeruginosa and S. aureus	Same as severe with risk factors, below
Severe (ICU admission, respiratory failure, rapid CXR progression, or sepsis with ↓BP and/or end organ dysfunction)	No risk factors AND hospitalized < 5 days	Same as mild to moderate, no risk factors
	No risk factors but hospitalized ≥5 days OR Risk factors for S. aureus, P. aeruginosa, or anaerobes	Vanco plus either Aminoglycoside, Cipro, Gati or Levo plus either: Pip/Tazo, Pip, Ticar/Clav, Imipenem, Meropenem, Aztreonam, or Cefepime

BAL=bronchoalveolar lavage, BOOP=bronchiolitis obliterans with organizing pneumonia. PBS=protected brush specimen, PE=pulmonary embolism, CHF=congestive heart failure. Aminoglycosides: adjust to level and renal function. Gentamicin or Tobramycin 3-5 mg/kg/d as single daily dose or divided into 2 or 3 doses. Amikacin 7.5mg/kg q12, not to exceed 1.5 g/day. Aztreonam 1g q8h-2g q6h, Azithromycin 500 mg qd, Cefepime 1.0-2.0 g q12h, Clinda=clindamycin 600 mg q8h, Cipro=ciprofloxacin 400-750 mg q12h, Gati = gatifloxacin 400 mg qd, Levo=levofloxacin 500 mg qd, Erythromycin 1.0g q6h, Nonpseudomonal 3rd gen Ceph=ceftriaxone 1-2 g qd, cefotaxime 2 g Q4-8, Pip/Tazo=piperacillin/tazobactam 3.375g q6h (antipseudomonal dose-4.5g q6h), Ticar/Clav=ticarcillin/clavulanate 3.1g q4-6h, Vanco=vancomycin 1.0g q12h, Pip=piperacillin 4g q6h, Imipenem 0.5 g q6h, Meropenem 0.5-1.0 g q8h

Hospital-acquired Pneumonia in Adults: Diagnosis, Assessment of Severity, Initial Antimicrobial Therapy, and Preventative Strategies. A Consensus Statement. Am J Respir Crit Care Med 153: 1711, 1996

3q: Pneumonia in the Immunocompromised Host

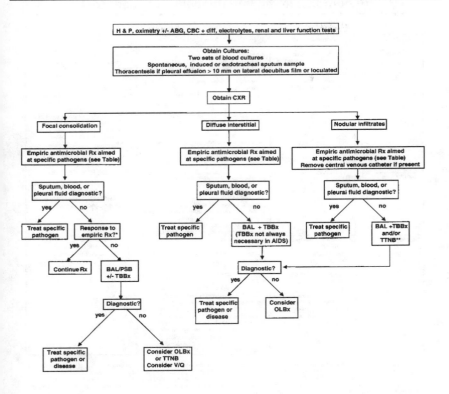

* If patient acutely ill and/or has a rapidly progressive process, may need to proceed directly to diagnostic procedure.
** TTNB especially useful if lesions are peripheral.

<u>Abbreviations</u>: BAL=bronchoalveolar lavage, PSB=protected specimen brush, TBBx =transbronchial biopsy, TTNB=transthoracic thin needle biopsy, V/Q=ventilation/perfusion scan, OLBx=open lung or thoracoscopic biopsy

Shelhamer, JH, moderator. NIH Conference: Respiratory disease in the immunocompromised patient. Ann Intern Med 117: 415, 1992

3r: Differential Diagnosis and Empiric Therapy for Pneumonia in the Immunocompromised Host

CXR Abnormality	Non-infectious Etiologies	Infectious Etiologies	Empiric Therapy
Focal Consolidation	Pulmonary embolism Pulmonary hemorrhage Tumor Less likely: Drug-induced Radiation-induced	**Bacterial** • Consider *S. pneumoniae*, *H. influenzae*, *Legionella pneumophila*, and *Mycoplasma pneumoniae* if acquired in community • Consider *S. aureus* and GNRs if acquired nosocomially Typical and atypical mycobacteria **Fungal:** *Aspergillus* species, *Histoplasma capsulatum*, *Cryptococcus neoformans*, *Coccidiodes immitis* *Nocardia asteroides* Less likely: *Pneumocystis carinii*, viral	**Community acquired:** • Macrolide ± 2nd gen ceph, non-pseudomonal 3rd gen ceph, Amp/Sulb, or "new" quinalone **Nosocomial:** • Non-pseudomonal 3rd gen ceph, Pip/Tazo, Ticar/Clav, imipenem, Meropenem, or combination of Clinda plus either Aztreonam, Gati, Levo, Cipro, Ceftazadine or Cefepime • Add Vanco if high incidence of MRSA • Add AG if severely ill • Add Ampho B if acutely ill and prolonged immunosupression and broad spectrum antibiotic use
Nodular Infiltrates	Tumor BOOP	Fungal: *Aspergillus* species, *Histoplasma capsulatum*, *Cryptococcus neoformans*, *Coccidiodes immitis* *Nocardia asteroides* Bacterial (especially septic emboli secondary to a central intravenous catheter) Typical and atypical mycobacteria Less likely: *Pneumocystis carinii*, *Legionella micdadei*, *Rhodococcus equi*	**Ampho B** Add Vanco + Gent if central venous catheter in place Consider TMP/S if severely ill while awaiting diagnostic evaluation

Diffuse Infiltrates	• Pulmonary edema
	• Drug-induced
	• Leukoagglutination reaction (Consider when syndrome occurs acutely following transfusion)
	• Radiation-induced
	• Tumor
	• Kaposis sarcoma (Consider in AIDS patient with skin or mucous membrane lesions)
	• Pulmonary hemorrhage
	• BOOP
		• *Pneumocystis carinii*
		• Viral
		  -Consider influenza if community acquired and appropriate season
		  -Consider CMV in transplant population. CMV only rarely a true pulmonary pathogen in AIDS
		  -Less common: VZV, HSV
		• Fungal: *Histoplasma capsulatum*, *Cryptococcus neoformans*
		• *Toxoplasma gondii*
		• Typical and atypical mycobacteria MTb commonly presents with diffuse infiltrates in advanced immunodeficiency
		• Bacterial: *Legionella pneumphila*, *Mycoplasma pneumoniae*, *Chlamydia pneumonia*
			TMP/S ± Macrolide
			Add Ganciclovir in transplant patients if appropriate risk factors are present

Abbreviations: GNR=gram negative rod, CMV=cytomegalovirus, VZV=varicella zoster virus, HSV=herpes simplex virus, MTb=*Mycobacterium tuberculosis*, BOOP=bronchiolitis obliterans with organizing pneumonia, Ceph=cephalosporin, Amp/Sulb=ampicillin/sulbactam, Pip/Tazo=piperacillin/tazobactam, Ticar/Clav=ticarcillin/clavulanate, Cipro = ciprofloxacin, Gati = gatifloxacin, Levo = levofloxacin, Clinda=clindamycin, Vanco=vancomycin, Pip=piperacillin, AG=aminoglycoside, Gent=gentamicin, TMP/S=trimethoprim sulfamethoxasole, Ampho B=amphotericin B

Reference: Shelhamer, JH, moderator. NIH Conference: Respiratory disease in the immunocompromised patient. Ann Intern Med 117: 415, 1992

3s: Tuberculosis Treatment

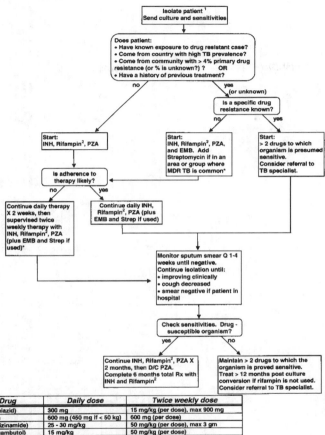

```
                    ┌─────────────────────────────┐
                    │ Isolate patient ¹            │
                    │ Send culture and sensitivities │
                    └─────────────────────────────┘
```

Isolate patient [1]
Send culture and sensitivities

Does patient:
• Have known exposure to drug resistant case?
• Come from country with high TB prevalence?
• Come from community with > 4% primary drug resistance (or % is unknown?) ?   **OR**
• Have a history of previous treatment?

→ **no**

→ **yes** (or unknown)

Is a specific drug resistance known?

→ **no**

→ **yes**

Start:
INH, Rifampin[2], PZA

Start:
INH, Rifampin[2], PZA, and EMB. Add Streptomycin if in an area or group where MDR TB is common*

Start:
> 2 drugs to which organism is presumed sensitive.
Consider referral to TB specialist.

Is adherence to therapy likely?

→ **no**

→ **yes**

Continue daily therapy X 2 weeks, then supervised twice weekly therapy with INH, Rifampin[2], PZA (plus EMB and Strep if used)*

Continue daily INH, Rifampin[2], PZA (plus EMB and Strep if used)

Monitor sputum smear Q 1-4 weeks until negative.
Continue isolation until:
• improving clinically
• cough decreased
• smear negative if patient in hospital

Check sensitivities. Drug - susceptible organism?

→ **yes**

→ **no**

Continue INH, Rifampin[2], PZA X 2 months, then D/C PZA. Complete 6 months total Rx with INH and Rifampin[2]

Maintain > 2 drugs to which the organism is proved sensitive. Treat > 12 months post culture conversion if rifampin is not used. Consider referral to TB specialist.

Drug	Daily dose	Twice weekly dose
INH (isoniazid)	300 mg	15 mg/kg (per dose), max 900 mg
Rifampin	600 mg (450 mg if < 50 kg)	600 mg (per dose)
PZA (pyrizinamide)	25 - 30 mg/kg	50 mg/kg (per dose), max 3 gm
EMB (ethambutol)	15 mg/kg	50 mg/kg (per dose)
Strep (streptomycin)	0.7-1.0 g	0.7-1.0 g (per dose)

1. Isolate in private room with negative airflow or recirculated through HEPA filter ± UV light source
2. Rifabutin 300 mg qd should be substituted for rifampin in HIV + receiving protease inhibitors or non-nucleoside reverse transcriptase inhibitors (NNRTIs). Rifabutin is contraindicated for use in pts taking certain antiretroviral Tx (consult 2nd ref. below, and/or TB specialist). See *Antiretroviral Agents* for listing of these agents.

ATS/CDC. Treatment of tuberculosis and tuberculosis infection in adults and children. Am Rev Respir Dis 149: 1359-1374; 1994
ATS/CDC. Targeted tuberculin testing and treatment of latent tuberculosis infection. Am J Respir Crit Care Med 161 (4 Pt 2): S221-47, 2000
Centers for Disease Control and Prevention. Prevention and treatment of TB among patients infected with HIV. MMWR 47(RR-20): 1-58, 1998

3t: Treatment of Latent Tuberculosis Infection (and Related Issues)

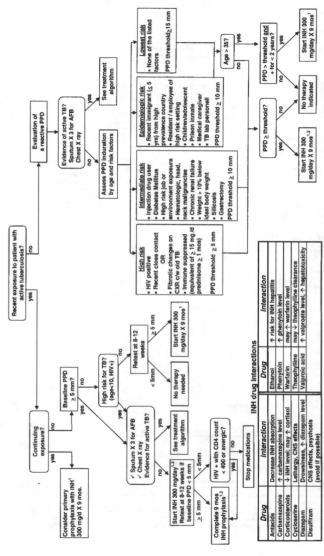

INH drug interactions

Drug	Interaction
Antacids	Decrease INH absorption
Carbamazepine	↑ carbamazepine level
Corticosteroids	↓ INH level; may ↑ cortisol
Cycloserine	Lethargy, CNS effects
Diazepam	Drowsiness, ↑ diazepam level
Disulfiram	CNS effects, psychosis (avoid if possible)

Drug	Interaction
Ethanol	↑ risk for INH hepatitis
Phenytoin	↑ phenytoin level
Warfarin	may ↑ warfarin level
Theophylline	may ↓ theophylline clearance
Valproic acid	↑ valproate level, ↑ hepatotoxicity

1. INH – Isoniazid. Monitor for adherence/side effects q 30d. Consider monthly LFTs if age >35 +/or liver disease, baseline LFTs abnormal, pregnant or immediately postpartum, INH interaction with other drugs possible (table), or "regular" ETOH use. Give pyridoxine (vitamin B6) 25-50 mg qd concommitantly to patients prone to neuropathy (ETOH abuse, diabetes).

2. A recently recommended alternative regimen for HIV – persons consists of daily rifampin 600 mg and PZA 25 mg/kg for 2 months. Rifabutin 300 mg qd should be substituted for rifampin in HIV + receiving protease inhibitors or non-nucleoside reverse transcriptase inhibitors (NNRTIs). Rifabutin is contraindicated for use in pts taking certain antiretroviral Tx (consult 2nd ref. below, and/or TB specialist). Monitor for adherence, drug interactions, side effects, LFTs CBC, platelets, weeks 2, 4, and 8. Treat hyperuricemia only if sx.

American Thoracic Society/Centers for Disease Control. Diagnostic standards and classification of tuberculosis in adults and children. Am J Respir Crit Care Med 161: 1376-1395, 2000
ATS/CDC Targeted tuberculin testing and treatment of latent tuberculosis infection. Am J Respir Crit Care Med 161 (4 Pt 2): S221-47, 2000
http://ajrccm.atsjournals.org/cgi/content/full/161/4/S1/S221
Centers for Disease Control and Prevention. Prevention and treatment of TB among patients infected with HIV. MMWR 47(RR-20): 1-58, 1998

4a: Diagnostic Algorithm for Hypotension and/or Shock

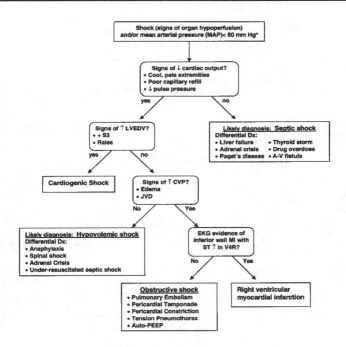

* MAP threshold is 75% of baseline value.

MAP – mean arterial pressure. LVEDV – left ventricular end diastolic volume. CVP – central venous pressure. JVD – jugular venous distension. MI – myocardial infarction. PEEP – positive end expiratory pressure. V4R – 4th right sided V lead

Hall JB et al. Principles of Critical Care 2nd ed., McGraw Hill, New York, 1998

4b: Therapeutic Algorithm for Hypotension and/or Shock

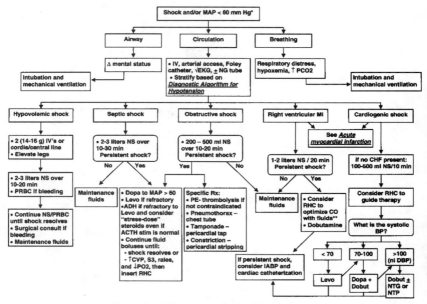

Shock and/or MAP < 60 mm Hg*

- **Airway** → Δ mental status → **Intubation and mechanical ventilation**
- **Circulation** → • IV, arterial access, Foley catheter, √EKG, ± NG tube • Stratify based on *Diagnostic Algorithm for Hypotension*
- **Breathing** → Respiratory distress, hypoxemia, ↑ PCO2 → **Intubation and mechanical ventilation**

Hypovolemic shock
- • 2 (14-16 g) IV's or cordis/central line • Elevate legs
- • 2-3 liters NS over 10-20 min • PRBC if bleeding
- • Continue NS/PRBC until shock resolves • Surgical consult if bleeding • Maintenance fluids

Septic shock
- • 2-3 liters NS over 10-30 min Persistent shock?
  - No → Maintenance fluids
  - Yes → • Dopa to MAP > 60 • Levo if refractory •ADH if refractory to Levo and consider "stress-dose" steroids even if ACTH stim is normal • Continue fluid boluses until: - shock resolves or - ↑CVP, S3, rales, and ↓PO2, then insert RHC

Obstructive shock
- • 200 – 500 ml NS over 10-20 min Persistent shock?
  - Yes → Specific Rx: • PE– thrombolysis if not contraindicated • Pneumothorax – chest tube • Tamponade – pericardial tap • Constriction – pericardial stripping
  - No → Maintenance fluids

If persistent shock, consider IABP and cardiac catheterization

Right ventricular MI → See *Acute myocardial infarction*
- 1-2 liters NS / 20 min Persistent shock?
  - No → Maintenance fluids
  - Yes → • Consider RHC to optimize CO with fluids** • Dobutamine

Cardiogenic shock → See *Acute myocardial infarction*
- If no CHF present: 100-500 ml NS/10 min
- Consider RHC to guide therapy
- What is the systolic BP?
  - < 70 → Levo
  - 70-100 → Dopa + Dobut
  - >100 (nl DBP) → Dobut ± NTG or NTP

**How to do a fluid challenge to maximize cardiac output

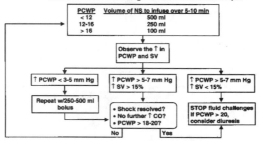

PCWP	Volume of NS to infuse over 5-10 min
< 12	500 ml
12-16	250 ml
> 16	100 ml

Observe the ↑ in PCWP and SV

- ↑ PCWP < 3-5 mm Hg → Repeat w/250-500 ml bolus
- ↑ PCWP > 5-7 mm Hg ↑ SV > 15% → • Shock resolved? • No further ↑ CO? • PCWP > 18-20?
  - No → (repeat) / Yes → STOP
- ↑ PCWP > 5-7 mm Hg ↑ SV < 15% → STOP fluid challenges If PCWP > 20, consider diuresis

---

Dopa – dopamine 2-20 mcg/kg/min; Dobut – dobutamine 5-15 mcg/kg/min; Levo – levophed 2-30 mcg/min; NTG – nitroglycerine 25-600 mcg/min
NTP – nitroprusside -0.1-5 mcg/kg/min; ADH– vasopressin 0.04-0.12 u/min. (*MAP goal is 75% of baseline value)
MAP – mean arterial pressure. DBP – diastolic blood pressure. RHC – right heart catheterization. SV – stroke volume (cardiac output/heart rate). NS – normal saline. PRBC – packed red blood cells. MI – myocardial infarction. IABP – intra-aortic balloon pump. CO – cardiac output.

Hall JB et al. Principles of Critical Care 2nd ed., McGraw Hill, New York, 1998
Guidelines for cardiopulmonary resuscitation and emergency cardiac care. JAMA 268: 2171, 1992
Malay MB et al. Low-dose vasopressin in the treatment of vasodilatory septic shock. J Trauma 47(4):699-703, 1999

4c: Table of Hemodynamic Subsets

Diagnosis	CVP	PCWP	CO	SVR	Comments
Hypovolemic Shock	↓	↓	↓	↑	
Distributive Shock (Sepsis, liver failure, thyroid storm, adrenal crisis, etc.)	nl or ↓	nl or ↓	nl or ↑	↓	May present with ↓ CO if under-resuscitated
Cardiogenic Shock					
Acute MI – predominantly LV	nl	↑	↓	↑	
Acute MI – predominantly RV	↑	nl or ↓	↓	↑	
Acute mitral regurgitation	nl or ↑	↑	↓	↑	• PCWP shows large V waves. • No step-up in O2 sats from RA to RV
Acute ventricular septal defect	nl or ↑	nl or ↑	↓*	↑	*measured CO by thermodilution or Fick method will overestimate CO if shunt is L to R. • Dx by step-up in O2 sats from RA to RV. • PCWP may show large V waves
Obstructive shock					
Massive pulmonary embolism	↑	nl or ↓	↓	↑	PAD >> PCWP; ↑ PVR
Pericardial tamponade	↑	↑	↓	↑	CVP ≅ PCWP; CVP shows loss of "y" descent
Tension pneumothorax	↑	↑	↓	↑	CVP ≅ PCWP
Occult autopeep	↑	↑	↓	↑	CVP ≅ PCWP. Suspect in patients with airway obstruction receiving assisted ventilation.

Normal values for hemodynamic parameters:

Central venous pressure (CVP):	2-8 mm Hg
Pulmonary capillary wedge pressure (PCWP):	5-12 mm Hg
Cardiac output (CO):	4-6 liters/min
Systemic vascular resistance (SVR):	900-1200 dyne-s/cm^5

PEEP – positive end expiratory pressure. MI – myocardial infarction. RA – right atrium. RV- right ventricle. LV – left ventricle. PAD – pulmonary artery diastolic pressure.

Hall JB et al. Principles of Critical Care 2nd ed., McGraw Hill, New York, 1998

4d: Management of Hypertensive Emergencies

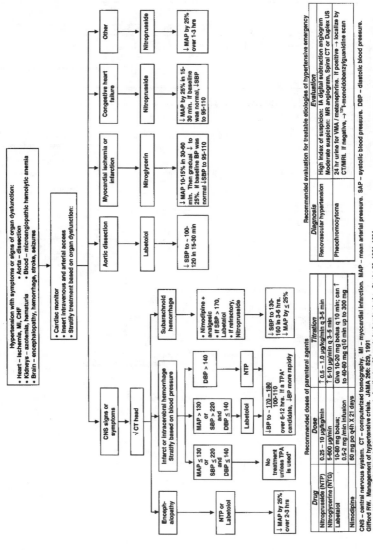

Hypertension with symptoms or signs of organ dysfunction:
- Heart – ischemia, MI, CHF
- Aorta – dissection
- Kidneys – azotemia, hematuria
- Blood – microangiopathic hemolytic anemia
- Brain – encephalopathy, hemorrhage, stroke, seizures

- Cardiac monitor
- Insert intravenous and arterial access
- Stratify treatment based on organ dysfunction:

Aortic dissection → Labetolol → ↓ SBP to ~ 100-120 in 15-30 min

Myocardial ischemia or infarction → Nitroglycerin → ↓ MAP 10-15% in 30-60 min. Then gradual ↓ to 25%. If baseline BP was normal ↓SBP to 95-110

Congestive heart failure → Nitroprusside → ↓ MAP by 25% in 15-30 min. If baseline BP was normal, ↓SBP to 95-110

Other → Nitroprusside → ↓ MAP by 25% over 1-3 hrs

CNS signs or symptoms

√ CT head

Encephalopathy → NTP or Labetolol → ↓ MAP by 25% over 2-3 hrs

Infarct or intracerebral hemorrhage
Stratify based on blood pressure

MAP ≤ 130 or SBP ≤ 220 and DBP ≤ 140 → No treatment unless TPA is used*

MAP > 130 or SBP > 220 and DBP ≤ 140 → Labetolol

DBP > 140 → NTP

↓BP to ~ 170 – 180 / 100-110 over 6-12 hrs. If a TPA* candidate, ↓BP more rapidly

Subarachnoid hemorrhage
- Nimodipine + analgesic
- If SBP > 170, Labetolol
- If refractory, Nitroprusside

↓ SBP to 130-160 in 3-6 hrs. ↓ MAP by ≤ 25%

Recommended doses of parenteral agents

Drug	Dose	Titration
Nitroprusside (NTP)	0.25 – 10 µg/kg/min	↑ 0.5 – 1.0 µg/kg/min q 3-5 min
Nitroglycerine (NTG)	5-600 µg/min	↑ 5-10 µg/min q 3-5 min
Labetolol	10-80 mg bolus; 0.5-2 mg /min infusion	Give 10-20 mg bolus q 10 min; can ↑ to 40-80 mg q10 min up to 300 mg
Nimodipine	60 mg po q4h X 21 days	

CNS – central nervous system. CT – computerized tomography. MI – myocardial infarction. MAP – mean arterial pressure. SAP – systemic blood pressure. DBP – diastolic blood pressure.
Gifford RW. Management of hypertensive crisis. JAMA 266: 829, 1991
Adams HA et al. Guidelines for the management of patients with acute ischemic stroke. Stroke 25: 1901, 1994
Brandt T et al. Neurologic Disorders: Course and Treatment, Academic Press, 1996

Recommended evaluation for treatable etiologies of hypertensive emergency

Diagnosis	Evaluation
Renovascular hypertension	High index of suspicion: IA digital subtraction angiogram. Moderate suspicion: MR angiogram, Spiral CT or Duplex US
Pheochromocytoma	24 hr urine for VMA / metanephrine. If positive → localize by CT/MRI. If negative, →[131I]-monoiodobenzylguanidine scan

* See Acute Stroke for TPA (tissue plasminogen activator) indications

4e: Ventilator Management

Indications for mechanical ventilation

Hypoxemia	Hypercapnia	Clinical
pO2 < 55 torr or SO2 < 92% despite supplemental inspired oxygen	pCO2 > 44 torr acutely; or pCO2 elevated chronically with pH < 7.25 despite non-invasive ventilation assist devices.	Respiratory distress accompanied by shock or somnolence.

Physician Orders:
Intubate patient: Oral ET tube size $\geq$ 7.0 (in adults) to avoid high airway resistance, suctioning difficulty, and possible occlusion from mucus and blood.

Initial Ventilator Settings:

Mode	Assist/Control (A/C*) or Intermittent Mandatory Ventilation (IMV*):
Inspired Oxygen (FIO2)	Select FIO2 based on PaO2 from previous ABG, or empirically start at FIO2 = 1.0 and decrease until SO2 = 94% (paO2 approximately 75 torr).
PEEP (cmH2O)	Begin at 5 to provide physiologic backpressure lost by the ET tube bypassing glottal muscles. Increase PEEP in increments of 2.5 to PEEP maximum* if the FIO2 $\geq$ 0.6.
Respiratory Rate (RR)	Begin at 8 – 12/min. Increase the RR if the patient's spontaneous RR > 6 above the set RR.
Tidal Volume (VT)	Patients without ARDS: Begin at 8 or 10 ml/KG and round off to the nearest 50 mL. Patients with ARDS: Use 6 ml/kg of ideal body weight
Nebulizer treatments	Albuterol, ipratropium bromide when indicated, frequency: at least q4h. See *COPD acute respiratory failure* and *Acute exacerbation of asthma.* Consider 2% bicarbonate solutions as mucolytic based on sputum viscosity.

Physician orders to adjust ventilator after initial settings and ABG:

Oxygenation (PO₂)

Adjust FIO2 and PEEP to alter SaO2.
↓
The SaO2 varies directly with the FIO2 and PEEP.
↓
For hypoxemia (SaO2 < 94%) requiring FIO2 > 0.6, first increase PEEP from 5 cm H2O in steps of 2.5 to a PEEP maximum*
↓
If hypoxemia persists, then increase the FIO2 in steps of 0.10 until 1.0 is reached or SO2>93%.
↓
For SO2 > 95% at PEEP maximum*, FIO2 is first reduced in steps of 0.10 until $\leq$ 0.6, then PEEP is reduced in steps of 2.5 to a minimum of 5 before further reductions of FIO2.

Ventilation (PCO₂)

Adjust RR and VT to alter pCO2 and pH.
↓
The pCO2 varies inversely with the VE* (RR x VT)

If pH < 7.35, increase VE (to lower pCO2) by increasing RR by 2/min to a maximum of 30; if acidemia persists, consider increasing VT in steps of 50 mL to maximum of 15mL/kg with the following caveats:
• In ARDS, high VT causes alveolar damage; Limit VT (~6 ml/kg ideal body weight) to keep plateau pressure $\leq$ 30. May allow permissive CO2 retention and lower pH.
• In COPD or asthma, high VE may cause autopeep. Autopeep should be measured before increasing VE. Aim for pH ~7.35, not for normal PCO2. In COPD or asthma, high VE may cause autopeep; minimize autopeep; keep plateau pressure < 30 and allow permissive CO2 retention.
↓
If pH > 7.45, decrease VE (to raise pCO2) by decreasing RR by 2 until $\leq$ 8, then decrease VT in steps of 50 mL.
If patient's RR remains elevated despite the ventilator RR reduction, consider sedation.

Pulmonary consultation should be considered for any patient on a ventilator and should be obtained for patients with ARDS or ventilatory failure due to any primary pulmonary disease state.

*Definitions:
A/C: Patient receives a set volume for every breath triggered by either patient effort (assist), or by time (control, based on the set Respiratory Rate).
IMV: Patient receives a set volume for the set Respiratory Rate, additional spontaneous breaths (non-set volume) can be taken at any time.
PEEP maximum: Positive End Expiratory Pressure (PEEP) producing improved oxygenation without significant compromise in hemodynamics, such as cardiac output, mixed venous saturation, and BP.
VE: Minute ventilation = Respiratory Rate x Tidal Volume
SaO2: Arterial oxygen saturation

ARDS Network. Ventilation with lower tidal volumes as compared with traditional tidal volumes for acute lung injury and the acute respiratory distress syndrome. N Engl J Med 342: 1301-1308, 2000
Branson RD. Monitoring ventilator function. Crit Care Clin 11:127-143, 1995.
Tobin MJ. Mechanical ventilation. N Engl J Med 330:1056-1061, 1994.
Hinson JR, Marinii JJ. Principles of mechanical ventilator use in respiratory failure. Ann Rev Med 43:341-361, 1992.

4f: Hypothermia

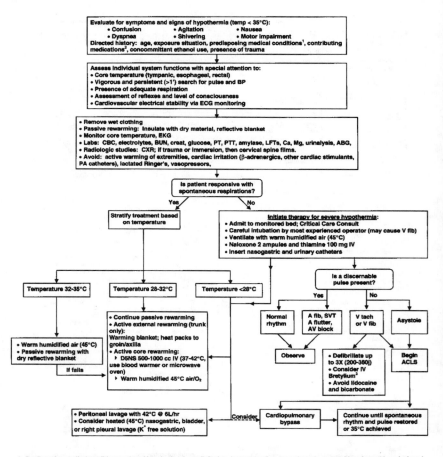

Evaluate for symptoms and signs of hypothermia (temp < 35°C):
- Confusion
- Agitation
- Nausea
- Dyspnea
- Shivering
- Motor Impairment

Directed history: age, exposure situation, predisposing medical conditions[1], contributing medications[2], concommittant ethanol use, presence of trauma

Assess individual system functions with special attention to:
- Core temperature (tympanic, esophageal, rectal)
- Vigorous and persistent (>1') search for pulse and BP
- Presence of adequate respiration
- Assessment of reflexes and level of consciousness
- Cardiovascular electrical stability via ECG monitoring

- Remove wet clothing
- Passive rewarming: Insulate with dry material, reflective blanket
- Monitor core temperature, EKG
- Labs: CBC, electrolytes, BUN, creat, glucose, PT, PTT, amylase, LFTs, Ca, Mg, urinalysis, ABG.
- Radiologic studies: CXR; if trauma or immersion, then cervical spine films.
- Avoid: active warming of extremities, cardiac irritation (β-adrenergics, other cardiac stimulants, PA catheters), lactated Ringer's, vasopressors.

Is patient responsive with spontaneous respirations?

Yes → **Stratify treatment based on temperature**

No → **Initiate therapy for severe hypothermia**
- Admit to monitored bed; Critical Care Consult
- Careful intubation by most experienced operator (may cause V fib)
- Ventilate with warm humidified air (45°C)
- Naloxone 2 ampules and thiamine 100 mg IV
- Insert nasogastric and urinary catheters

Is a discernable pulse present?

Yes / No

Temperature 32-35°C
- Warm humidified air (45°C)
- Passive rewarming with dry reflective blanket

If fails

Temperature 28-32°C
- Continue passive rewarming
- Active external rewarming (trunk only):
Warming blanket; heat packs to groin/axilla
- Active core rewarming:
  ‣ D5NS 500-1000 cc IV (37-42°C, use blood warmer or microwave oven)
  ‣ Warm humidified 45°C air/O2

Temperature <28°C

(Yes) Normal rhythm → Observe

A fib, SVT A flutter, AV block → Observe

(No) V tach or V fib
- Defibrillate up to 3X (200-360j)
- Consider IV Bretylium[3]
- Avoid lidocaine and bicarbonate

Asystole → Begin ACLS

- Peritoneal lavage with 42°C @ 6L/hr
- Consider heated (45°C) nasogastric, bladder, or right pleural lavage (K+ free solution)

← Consider → **Cardiopulmonary bypass**

Continue until spontaneous rhythm and pulse restored or 35°C achieved

1. Predisposing medical conditions: ethanol intoxication, hypopituitarism, hypoadrenalism, hypoglycemia, malnutrition, dermatitis, spinal cord injury, diabetes, CNS lesion, sepsis, uremia, Paget's disease
2. Contributing medications: ethanol, phenothiazines, benzodiazepines, antidepressants, barbiturates, narcotics, clonidine
3. Bretylium tosylate 5-10mg/kg loading dose, 1-2 mg/min maintenance dose. Procainamide should be avoided.

Weinberg A. Hypothermia. Ann Emerg Med 22:370-377, 1933
Gentilello L. Advances in the management of hypothermia. Surg Clin zNA 75:243-256, 1995
Danzi DF, Pozos RS. Accidental hypothermia. N Engl J Med 331: 1756-1760, 1994
Lazar HL. The treatment of hypothermia. N Engl J Med 337: 1545 – 47, 1997

4g: Hyperthermia

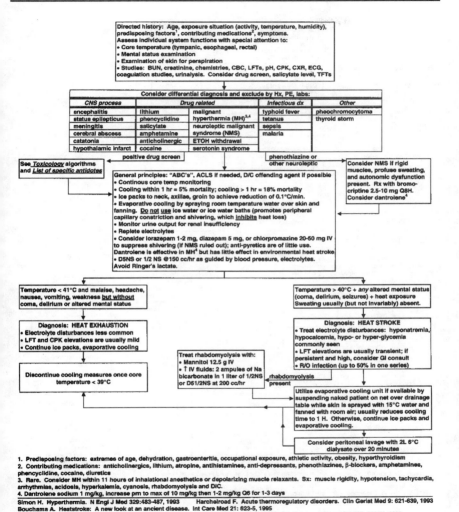

Directed history: Age, exposure situation (activity, temperature, humidity), predisposing factors[1], contributing medications[2], symptoms.
Assess individual system functions with special attention to:
- Core temperature (tympanic, esophageal, rectal)
- Mental status examination
- Examination of skin for perspiration
- Studies: BUN, creatinine, chemistries, CBC, LFTs, pH, CPK, CXR, ECG, coagulation studies, urinalysis. Consider drug screen, salicylate level, TFTs

Consider differential diagnosis and exclude by Hx, PE, labs:

CNS process	Drug related		Infectious dx	Other
encephalitis	lithium	malignant	typhoid fever	pheochromocytoma
status epilepticus	phencyclidine	hyperthermia (MH)[3,4]	tetanus	thyroid storm
meningitis	salicylate	neuroleptic malignant	sepsis	
cerebral abscess	amphetamine	syndrome (NMS)	malaria	
catatonia	anticholinergic	ETOH withdrawal		
hypothalamic infarct	cocaine	serotonin syndrome		

See *Toxicology* algorithms and *List of specific antidotes* ← positive drug screen

phenothiazine or other neuroleptic →

Consider NMS if rigid muscles, profuse sweating, and autonomic dysfunction present. Rx with bromocriptine 2.5-10 mg Q8H. Consider dantrolene[4]

General principles: "ABC's", ACLS if needed, D/C offending agent if possible
- Continous core temp monitoring
- Cooling within 1 hr = 5% mortality; cooling > 1 hr = 18% mortality
- Ice packs to neck, axillae, groin to achieve reduction of 0.1°C/min.
- Evaporative cooling by spraying room temperature water over skin and fanning. Do not use ice water or ice water baths (promotes peripheral capillary constriction and shivering, which inhibits heat loss)
- Monitor urine output for renal insufficiency
- Replete electrolytes
- Consider lorazepam 1-2 mg, diazepam 5 mg, or chlorpromazine 20-50 mg IV to suppress shivering (if NMS ruled out); anti-pyretics are of little use.
Dantrolene is effective in MH[4] but has little effect in environmental heat stroke
- D5NS or 1/2 NS @150 cc/hr as guided by blood pressure, electrolytes.
Avoid Ringer's lactate.

Temperature < 41°C and malaise, headache, nausea, vomiting, weakness but without coma, delirium or altered mental status

Diagnosis: HEAT EXHAUSTION
- Electrolyte disturbances less common
- LFT and CPK elevations are usually mild
- Continue ice packs, evaporative cooling

Discontinue cooling measures once core temperature < 39°C

Treat rhabdomyolysis with:
- Mannitol 12.5 g IV
- ↑ IV fluids: 2 ampules of Na bicarbonate in 1 liter of 1/2NS or D51/2NS at 200 cc/hr

Temperature > 40°C + any altered mental status (coma, delirium, seizures) + heat exposure Sweating usually (but not invariably) absent.

Diagnosis: HEAT STROKE
- Treat electrolyte disturbances: hyponatremia, hypocalcemia, hypo- or hyper-glycemia commonly seen
- LFT elevations are usually transient; if persistent and high, consider GI consult
- R/O infection (up to 50% in one series)

rhabdomyolysis present →

Utilize evaporative cooling unit if available by suspending naked patient on net over drainage table while skin is sprayed with 15°C water and fanned with room air; usually reduces cooling time to 1 H. Otherwise, continue ice packs and evaporative cooling.

Consider peritoneal lavage with 2L 6°C dialysate over 20 minutes

1. **Predisposing factors:** extremes of age, dehydration, gastroenteritis, occupational exposure, athletic activity, obesity, hyperthyroidism
2. **Contributing medications:** anticholinergics, lithium, atropine, antihistamines, anti-depressants, phenothiazines, β-blockers, amphetamines, phencyclidine, cocaine, diuretics
3. **Rare.** Consider MH within 11 hours of inhalational anesthetics or depolarizing muscle relaxants. Sx: muscle rigidity, hypotension, tachycardia, arrhythmias, acidosis, hyperkalemia, cyanosis, rhabdomyolysis and DIC.
4. **Dantrolene sodium** 1 mg/kg, increase prn to max of 10 mg/kg then 2 mg/kg Q6 for 1-3 days

Simon H. Hyperthermia. N Engl J Med 329:483-487, 1993   Harchelroad F. Acute thermoregulatory disorders. Clin Geriat Med 9: 621-639, 1993
Bouchama A. Heatstroke: A new look at an ancient disease. Int Care Med 21: 623-5, 1995
Yaqub B, Aldeeb S. Heatstroke: etiopathogenesis, neurological characteristics, treatment and outcome. J Neurol Sci 136: 144-51, 1998

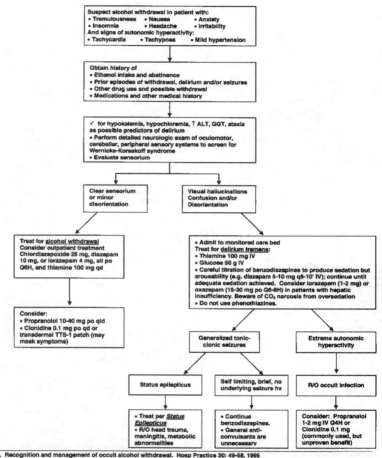

Suspect alcohol withdrawal in patient with:
- Tremulousness • Nausea • Anxiety
- Insomnia • Headache • Irritability

And signs of autonomic hyperactivity:
- Tachycardia • Tachypnea • Mild hypertension

Obtain history of
- Ethanol intake and abstinence
- Prior episodes of withdrawal, delirium and/or seizures
- Other drug use and possible withdrawal
- Medications and other medical history

✓ for hypokalemia, hypochloremia, ↑ ALT, GGT, ataxia as possible predictors of delirium
- Perform detailed neurologic exam of oculomotor, cerebellar, peripheral sensory systems to screen for Wernicke-Korsakoff syndrome
- Evaluate sensorium

Clear sensorium or minor disorientation

Visual hallucinations Confusion and/or Disorientation

Treat for alcohol withdrawal
Consider outpatient treatment
Chlordiazepoxide 25 mg, diazepam 10 mg, or lorazepam 4 mg, all po Q6H, and thiamine 100 mg qd

- Admit to monitored care bed
Treat for delirium tremens:
- Thiamine 100 mg IV
- Glucose 50 g IV
- Careful titration of benzodiazepines to produce sedation but arousability (e.g. diazepam 5-10 mg q5-10' IV); continue until adequate sedation achieved. Consider lorazepam (1-2 mg) or oxazepam (15-30 mg po Q6-8H) in patients with hepatic insufficiency. Beware of CO_2 narcosis from oversedation
- Do not use phenothiazines.

Consider:
- Propranolol 10-40 mg po qid
- Clonidine 0.1 mg po qd or transdermal TTS-1 patch (may mask symptoms)

Generalized tonic-clonic seizures

Extreme autonomic hyperactivity

Status epilepticus

Self limiting, brief, no underlying seizure hx

R/O occult infection

- Treat per Status Epilepticus
- R/O head trauma, meningitis, metabolic abnormalities

- Continue benzodiazepines.
- General anti-convulsants are unnecessary

Consider: Propranolol 1-2 mg IV Q4H or Clonidine 0.1 mg (commonly used, but unproven benefit)

Saltz R. Recognition and management of occult alcohol withdrawal. Hosp Practice 30: 49-58, 1995
Mayo-Smith M. Pharmacological management of alcohol withdrawal: A meta-analysis and evidence based practice guidelines. JAMA 278: 144-51, 1997
Hall W, Zador D. The alcohol withdrawal syndrome. Lancet 349: 1897 – 1900, 1997

4i: Equations

Conversions

Weight:

1kg = 2.2 lbs	1 lb = 0.454 kg	1 ounce = 30 g
1 tspn = 5 ml	1 tbspn = 15 ml	1 ounce = 30 ml

Temperature

$$°F = 32 + 9/5(°C) \qquad °C = 5/9(°F - 32)$$

1 inch = 2.54 cm   1 cm = 0.3973 inch

$BSA (m^2) = [((ht(cm) \times wt(kg))/3600]^{0.5}$

Ventilation

$PAO_2 = FIO_2((Pb-47)-PCO_2/R$
A-a gradient = PAO2 – measured PaO2 (from blood gas)
age correction for "normal" O2 = 100 - 1/3 (age)
$PACO_2 = (0.863 \times VCO_2)/V_A$
Oxygen content (C)= $(1.36 \times Hb \times \%Sat) + 0.003(PO_2)$
$Qs/Qt = [(Cc'O_2 - CaO_2)/(Cc'O_2 - CvO_2)] \times 100$
Qs/Qt estimate: (A-a gradient on 100%)/16
Compliance = VT/(Pplateau - peep)
Resistance = 60 × (Ppleak - Pplateau) /Flow
$V_D/V_T = (PaCO_2 - PeCO_2)/PaCO_2$

P - partial pressure (A - alveolar, a - arterial, e - mixed expired); FIO2 - fraction of inspired O2; R - respiratory exchange ratio (~0.8); V_A - minute alveolar ventilation; V_D/V_T - dead space /tidal volume ratio; c' - end capillary, v - mixed venous

Hemodynamics

Mean arterial pressure (MAP)= (1/3)systolic + (2/3)diastolic
Fick equation: Cardiac output (CO) = 10 × VO_2/CaO_2 - CvO_2
Systemic vascular resistance (SVR) = [(MAP - mRAP) × 80]/CO
Pulmonary vascular resistance (PVR) = [(mPAP -PCW) × 80]/CO
Oxygen delivery (DO2) = CO × 1.36 × Hb × SaO_2
Cerebral Perfusion Pressure = MAP - ICP

mRAP - mean right atrial pressure; mPAP - mean pulmonary artery pressure; PCW - pulmonary artery occlusion pressure

Acid Base Disorders (See _Renal_ section)

Acute respiratory acidosis:	$\Delta pH = 0.008(\Delta PCO_2)$
Chronic respiratory acidosis:	$\Delta pH = 0.003(\Delta PCO_2)$
Acute respiratory alkalosis:	$\Delta pH = 0.008(\Delta PCO_2)$
Chronic respiratory alkalosis:	$\Delta pH = 0.002(\Delta PCO_2)$

Anion gap = Na - (Cl + HCO3)   Normal < 10-14; AG will decrease by 2.5 for every 1 g/dl decrease in albumin

Nutrition (see _Nutrition equations_ and _Nutrition_ section)

Harris - Benedict equations: Males: REE = 66.47 + 13.75(IBW) + 5.0H - 6.76A
   Females: REE = 655.1 + 9.5(IBW) + 9.56H - 4.68A
Sherman equation   MEE = 9.27 $(P_ECO_2)(V_E)$
Ligget - St. John - LeFrak equation   MEE = 95.18 (CO) (Hb) (SaO_2-SvO_2)
Nitrogen balance = Protein intake(g)/6.25 - (24 hr UUN(g) + 4)

REE – resting energy expenditure. MEE – measured energy expenditure. IBW – ideal body weight (kg). H – height (cm). A – age (years). CO - cardiac output. P_ECO_2 partial pressure of expired CO_2 (collect 2-5 liters mixed expired gas, remove 10 ml and inject through blood gas analyzer). SaO_2 and SvO_2 saturations must be measured by co-oximetry. VE – minute ventilation. UUN – urinary urea nitrogen

Renal/Fluid and electrolytes

Total body water = 0.6 × lean body weight (kg) (males); = 0.5 × lean body weight (kg) (females)
Estimation of lean/ideal body weight: females: =45.5 kg for first 5', then 2.3 kg each additional inch
   males: =48 kg for first 5', then 2.7 kg each additional inch

Creatinine clearance (CCL):
     Measured = (urine Cr (mg/dl) × total volume (ml)/[serum Cr (mg/dl)× time(min)]
     Cockcroft-Gault formula : CCL = [(140-age) × weight(kg)/72 × serum Cr] × (0.85 if female obese or edema)
     Age based estimate: CCL = [100-(age-30)]/serum Cr
Cl^- deficit = 0.5(wt in kg)(103-serum Cl^- (meq))
Na deficit = 0.6 (wt in kg)(140 - Na)+ 140(H_2O deficit in l)
H_2O deficit = 0.6 (wt in kg)(Na/140 - 1)
Calculated osmolality = 2(Na) + (glucose/18) + (BUN/2.8) + (mannitol/18) + (EtOH/4.6)
Osmolar gap = actual osmolality - calculated. Normal range: 0-5.
FeNa = (Urine Na/Plasma Na)/(Urine Creatinine/Plasma Creatinine). FeNa < 1 is prerenal
Na correction for high glucose: Actual Na = measured Na + 1.6 × [(measured glucose - 100)/100]
Ca correction for low albumin: Corrected Ca = measured Ca + 0.8 (4.0 - measured albumin)
Cr = creatinine.

5a: Dysphagia

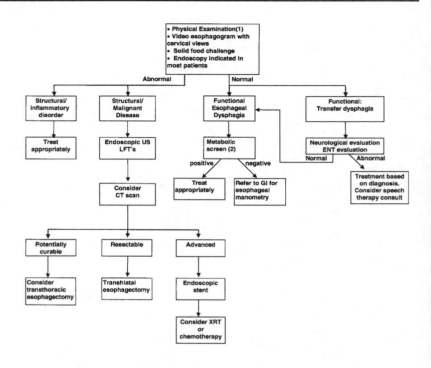

(1) Physical exam: Should include detailed oropharyngeal, head and neck exam, exam of cervical and supraclavicular lymph nodes, and a detailed neurologic exam with focus on cranial nerves, speech and frontal release signs.

(2) Metabolic screen: includes erythrocyte sedimentation rate, ANA, Jo, Ku, Mi antigens (polymyositis), SCL-70 (scleroderma), anti-centromere antibody (CREST), ANA and double stranded DNA Ab (SLE), fasting glucose, thyroid studies (myxedma). Consider biopsy for amyloidosis during endoscopy.

5b: Management of Peptic Ulcer Disease

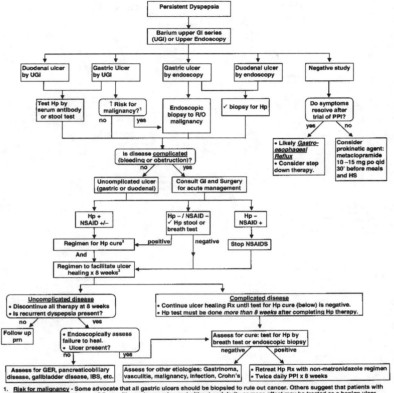

1. **Risk for malignancy** - Some advocate that all gastric ulcers should be biopsied to rule out cancer. Others suggest that patients with NSAID use, small antral ulcers, < 0.5 cm with regular margins and without nodularity or mass effect may be treated as a benign ulcer without endoscopy. Such patients not biopsied should have complete ulcer healing documented by repeat barium study.

2. **Regimens for Hp cure** (This is not a complete list. Regimens change rapidly and current regimens should be sought)
- Metronidazole 250 mg PO QID, Tetracycline 500 mg PO QID, Bismuth subsalicylate 2 tablets PO QID, Ranitidine 150 mg bid (14 day) OR
- Metronidazole 500 mg PO BID, Clarithromycin 500 mg PO BID, Omeprazole 20 mg PO BID (7 day) OR
- Amoxicillin 1000 mg PO BID, Clarithromycin 500 mg PO BID, Omeprazole 20 mg PO BID (7 day) OR
- Tritec (ranitadine/ bismuth combination) bid, metronidazole 500 mg bid, clarithromycin 500 mg bid (7 day)

3. **Regimens to facilitate ulcer healing** (oral doses given)
PPI (Proton pump inhibitor): Omeprazole 20 mg QD, Lansoprazole 30 mg QD, Rabeprazalole 20 mg QD, Pantoprazole 40 mg QD
H2 receptor antagonist: Cimetidine 400 mg BID, Ranitidine 150 mg BID, Famotidine 20 mg BID, Nizatidine 150 mg BID
Other: Sucralfate 1 gram QID

Abbreviations: Hp = Helicobacter pylori, NSAID = Non-steroidal anti-inflammatory drug, IBS = irritable bowel syndrome

Soll, A. H. Medical treatment of Peptic Ulcer Disease: Practice guidelines. JAMA; 275:622 1996
Isenberg, J.I. et al. Acid-Peptic Disorders. In Textbook of Gastroenterology, 2nd edition. T.Yamada ed. Lippincott Co., Philadelphia. 1996.
Peterson et al. Helicobacter pylori-related disease: guidelines for testing and treatment. Arch Intern Med. 2000 May 8;160(9):1285-91

5c: Gastroesophageal Reflux

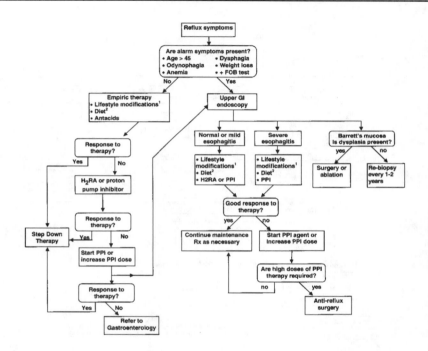

[1] Lifestyle modification:
- Do not lie down for 2 hours post prandial
- Elevate head of bed 4 to 6 inches
- Stop smoking

[2] Diet   Avoid fatty foods, eating late, large meals, onions, spaghetti sauce, chocolate, soda, coffee

FOB – fecal occult blood
H2RA – Histamine-2 receptor blockers:
    Cimetidine 300 mg po bid or Famotidine 20 mg bid or Nizatadine 150 mg po bid or Ranitidine 150 mg po bid
PPI – Protein pump inhibitors:
    Omeprazole 20 mg or Lansoprazole 30 mg or Rabeprazole 20 mg or Pantoprazole 40 mg po or Eisonmeprazole 40 mg qAM before breakfast

DiPalma JA. Management of severe gastroesophageal reflux disease. J Clin Gastroenterol 2001 Jan;32(1):19-26
Spechler SJ. Barrett's Esophagus. The Gastroenterologist, 1994: 2: 273-84
Devault KR. Current Management of gastroesophageal reflux disease. The Gastroenterologist 1996; 4: 24-32

5d: Approach to the Patient with Acute Diarrhea

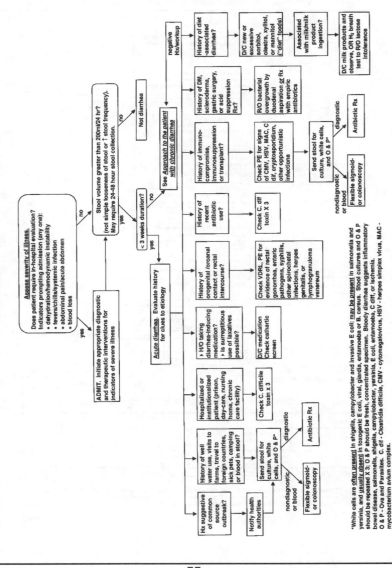

Assess severity of illness.
Does patient require in-hospital evaluation?
Indicators prompting admission (any one):
• dehydration/hemodynamic instability
• fevers/chills/systemic infection
• abdominal pain/acute abdomen
• blood loss

ADMIT. Initiate appropriate diagnostic and therapeutic interventions for indicators of severe illness.

Stool volume greater than 200ml/24 hr?
(not simple looseness of stool or ↑ stool frequency).
May require 24-48 hour stool collection.

Not diarrhea

See *Approach to the patient with chronic diarrhea*

< 3 weeks duration?

Acute diarrhea. Evaluate history for clues to etiology.

Hx suggestive of common source outbreak?

Notify health authorities

History of well water use, visits to farms, travel to foreign countries, sick pets, camping or blood in stool?

Hospitalized or institutionalized patient (prison, day-care, nursing home, chronic care facility)

Check C. difficile toxin x 3

Send stool for culture, white cells, and O & P*

Flexible sigmoid- or colonoscopy

Antibiotic Rx

↑ H/O taking diarrhea-inducing medication?
↑ Is surreptitious use of laxatives possible?

D/C medication
Check cathartic screen

History of orogenital /oroanal contact or rectal intercourse?

Check VDRL, PE for evidence of rectal gonorrhea, syphilis, other spirochetal infections, herpes genitalis, or lymphogranuloma venereum

History of recent antibiotic use?

Check C. diff toxin X 3

History of immunocompromise, immunosuppression or transplant?

Check PE for signs of CMV, HSV, MAC, C diff, cryptosporidium, other opportunistic infections

Send stool for culture, white cells, and O & P*

Flexible sigmoid- or colonoscopy

Antibiotic Rx

History of DM, scleroderma, gastric surgery, or acid suppression Rx?

R/O bacterial overgrowth by duodenal aspiration or Rx with empiric antibiotics

negative Hx/workup

History of diet -associated diarrhea?

D/C new or excessive sorbitol, olestra, xylitol, or mannitol ("diet" foods)

Associated with milk/milk product ingestion?

D/C milk products and observe, OR H₂ breath test to R/O lactose intolerance

*White cells are often present in shigella, campylobacter and invasive E coli; may be present in salmonella and yersinia, and usually absent in toxogenic E coli, viral, giardia, entamoeba or B. cereus. Stool cultures and O & P should be repeated X 3; O & P should be fresh, concentrated specimen. Bloody diarrhea suggests inflammatory bowel disease, salmonella, shigella, campylobacter, yersinia, E coli, entamoeba, C diff, or ischemia. O & P - Ova and Parasites. C. diff - Clostridia difficile, CMV - cytomegalovirus, HSV - herpes simplex virus, MAC - mycobacterium avium complex.

5e: Approach to the Patient with Chronic Diarrhea

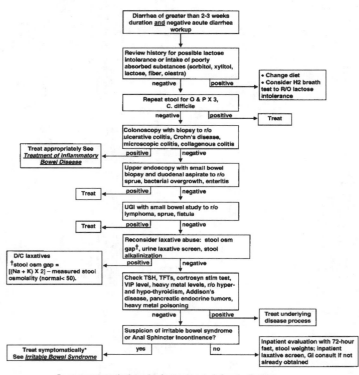

Class	Drug	Dose
Antisecretory	Bismuth subsalicylate	2 tabs every 30-60 minutes to maximum of 8 doses/24 hours
Adsorbent	Attapulgite (Donnagel, Diasorb, Kaopectate, Parepectolin,)	As directed
Opiates	Lomotil (diphenoxylate/atropine) Imodium (loperamide) Tincture of opium	up to 2 tabs qid 4 mg(2tabs) 3-6 drops q 6 hours
Adrenergic blockers	Clonidine	0.1 mg - 0.3 mg po q 8 hours

*Some symptomatic therapies for treatment of chronic diarrhea

Donowitz M, Kokke FT, Saidi R. Evaluation of patients with chronic diarrhea. New England Journal of Medicine 332(11):725-9, 1995.
Powell DS Approach to the patient with diarrhea. In: Yamada T, ed. Textbook of Gastroenterology. Philadelphia: J.B. Lippincott, 1995: 813-831.
Fine KD. Diarrhea. In: Feldman: Sleisenger & Fordtran's Gastrointestinal and Liver Disease, Sixth Edition. Philadelphia, W. B. Saunders Company, 1998: 128-149.

5f: Constipation

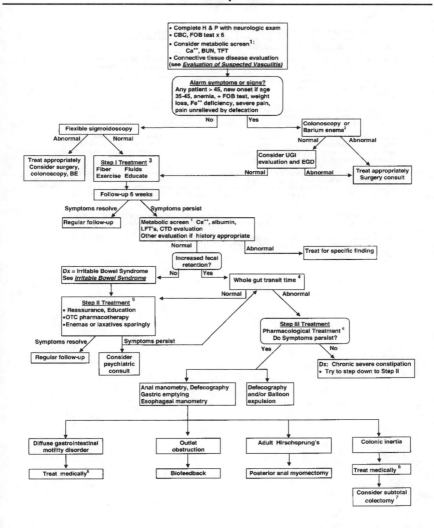

- Complete H & P with neurologic exam
- CBC, FOB test x 5
- Consider metabolic screen[1]:
  Ca++, BUN, TFT
- Connective tissue disease evaluation
  (see *Evaluation of Suspected Vasculitis*)

Alarm symptoms or signs?
Any patient > 45, new onset if age 35-45, anemia, + FOB test, weight loss, Fe++ deficiency, severe pain, pain unrelieved by defecation

No → **Yes**

No: Flexible sigmoidoscopy

Yes: Colonoscopy or Barium enema[2]
- Normal
- Abnormal

Normal → Consider UGI evaluation and EGD → Normal / Abnormal

Abnormal (Colonoscopy) → Treat appropriately, Surgery consult

Flexible sigmoidoscopy
- Abnormal → Treat appropriately, Consider surgery, colonoscopy, BE
- Normal → **Step I Treatment**[3]
  Fiber   Fluids
  Exercise Educate

Follow-up 5 weeks
- Symptoms resolve → Regular follow-up
- Symptoms persist → Metabolic screen[1] Ca++, albumin, LFT's, CTD evaluation. Other evaluation if history appropriate
  - Normal
  - Abnormal → Treat for specific finding

Increased fecal retention?
- No → Dx = Irritable Bowel Syndrome. See *Irritable Bowel Syndrome*
- Yes → **Whole gut transit time**[4]
  - Normal
  - Abnormal

Step II Treatment[5]
- Reassurance, Education
- OTC pharmacotherapy
- Enemas or laxatives sparingly

- Symptoms resolve → Regular follow-up
- Symptoms persist → Consider psychiatric consult

Step III Treatment
Pharmacological Treatment[6]
Do Symptoms persist?
- Yes
- No → Dx: Chronic severe constipation. Try to step down to Step II

Yes:
- Anal manometry, Defecography, Gastric emptying, Esophageal manometry
- Defecography and/or Balloon expulsion

- Diffuse gastrointestinal motility disorder → Treat medically[5]
- Outlet obstruction → Biofeedback
- Adult Hirschsprung's → Posterior anal myomectomy
- Colonic inertia → Treat medically[6] → Consider subtotal colectomy[7]

5f: Constipation (continued)

1. Metabolic screen should include: fasting glucose, thyroid function tests, calcium and electrolytes. In selected patients consider: amylase, heavy metal poisoning (especially lead) and connective tissue serologies (see *Evaluation of Suspected Vasculitis* and *Interpretation of Positive Fluorescent Antinuclear Antibody Test*).

2. Barium enema is most useful in the evaluation of rectocele, rectal prolapse, or extrinsic lesions: endometriosis, neoplasms (ovarian, prostate, renal, mesenteric, lymphoma), severe stricture, and large uterine fibroid.

3. Step I Treatment: Non-pharmacologic treatment: Stop aggravating medications, 25-30 gram high-fiber diet, exercise, fluids, bowel retraining, and patient education. Often useful to initiate these treatments after bowel cleansing with tap water enemas or osmotic laxatives.

4. Whole Gut Transit Time: Several techniques available. Least expensive (and also highly effective) is the radio-opaque marker study. Patient swallows 20 radio-opaque plastic markers. Abdominal x-ray (KUB) is taken 3 hours and 4 days later. 80% of markers should be eliminated after 4 days. If markers are present, another x-ray on day 7 may confirm severity.

5. Step II Treatment: Non-prescription therapy: If constipation persists, add over-the-counter laxatives to Step I treatment. Minimize the use of contact (irritant) laxatives (e.g. Ex-Lax®). Osmotic, magnesium based salts are safe when used sparingly. They cannot be used in patients with renal failure. Intermittent purging with contact laxatives or tap water enemas may prevent excessive distention of bowel loops.

6. Step III Treatment: Pharmacologic Treatment: Emphasize safety, low cost and efficacy. Use osmotic laxatives including Milk of Magnesia, saline or balanced PEG solutions. Avoid habitual use of laxatives or enemas, although their judicious use is helpful. Avoid agents that increase bloating/gas: carbonated beverages, gaseous foods, poorly absorbed carbohydrates (lactulose, sorbitol, lactose). New prokinetic agents (5HT4 agonists) effective in the lower GI tract should be considered when FDA approved.

7. Subtotal Colectomy: Recommended in highly selected patients who have normal upper GI motility and normal psychological status. Procedure of choice is a subtotal colectomy, ileo-rectal anastomosis. Very rarely necessary.

FOB test: fecal occult blood test; PEG: polyethylene glycol (e.g. Colyte, Golytely, Nulytlely 4-8 oz QOD, increase as needed). Some authors recommend 1 liter consumed once weekly.

5g: Irritable Bowel Syndrome

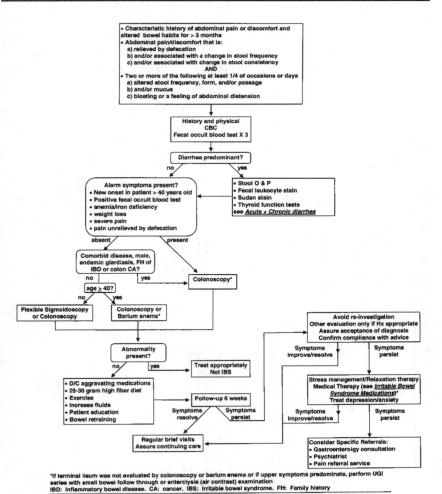

- Characteristic history of abdominal pain or discomfort and altered bowel habits for > 3 months
- Abdominal pain/discomfort that is:
  a) relieved by defecation
  b) and/or associated with a change in stool frequency
  c) and/or associated with change in stool consistency
  AND
- Two or more of the following at least 1/4 of occasions or days
  a) altered stool frequency, form, and/or passage
  b) and/or mucus
  c) bloating or a feeling of abdominal distension

↓

History and physical
CBC
Fecal occult blood test X 3

↓

Diarrhea predominant?

no → yes

yes:
- Stool O & P
- Fecal leukocyte stain
- Sudan stain
- Thyroid function tests
see *Acute + Chronic diarrhea*

no:
Alarm symptoms present?
- New onset in patient > 40 years old
- Positive fecal occult blood test
- anemia/iron deficiency
- weight loss
- severe pain
- pain unrelieved by defecation

absent / present

absent:
Comorbid disease, male, endemic giardiasis, FH of IBD or colon CA?

no / yes

present → Colonoscopy*

no (comorbid): age ≥ 40?

no / yes

no: Flexible Sigmoidoscopy or Colonoscopy
yes: Colonoscopy or Barium enema*

↓

Abnormality present?

no / yes

yes: Treat appropriately
Not IBS

no:
- D/C aggravating medications
- 25-30 gram high fiber diet
- Exercise
- Increase fluids
- Patient education
- Bowel retraining

→ Follow-up 6 weeks

Symptoms resolve / Symptoms persist

Symptoms resolve: Regular brief visits
Assure continuing care

Symptoms persist → Stress management/Relaxation therapy
Medical Therapy (see *Irritable Bowel Syndrome Medications*)*
Treat depression/anxiety

Symptoms improve/resolve / Symptoms persist

Avoid re-investigation
Other evaluation only if Hx appropriate
Assure acceptance of diagnosis
Confirm compliance with advice

Symptoms improve/resolve / Symptoms persist

Symptoms persist → Consider Specific Referrals:
- Gastroenterology consultation
- Psychiatrist
- Pain referral service

*If terminal ileum was not evaluated by colonoscopy or barium enema or if upper symptoms predominate, perform UGI series with small bowel follow through or enterclysis (air contrast) examination
IBD: Inflammatory bowel disease. CA: cancer. IBS: Irritable bowel syndrome. FH: Family history

Longstreth GF. Irritable bowel syndrome. Diagnosis in the managed care era. Dig Dis Sci 1997; 42:1105-11
Farthing MJ. Irritable bowel, irritable body, or irritable brain? BMJ 310; 1995: 171-5

5h: Irritable Bowel Syndrome Medications

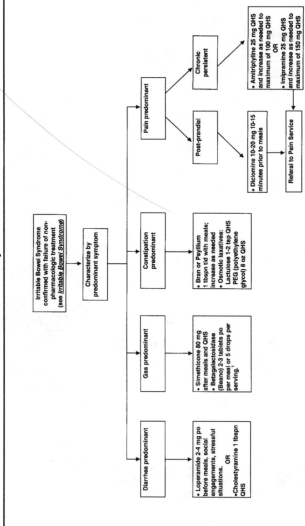

Irritable Bowel Syndrome confirmed with failure of non-pharmacologic treatment (see *Irritable Bowel Syndrome*)

↓

Characterize by predominant symptom

Diarrhea predominant
- Loperamide 2-4 mg po before meals, social engagements, stressful situations.
  OR
- Cholestyramine 1 tbspn QHS

Gas predominant
- Simethicone 80 mg after meals and QHS
- Betagalactosidase (Beano) 2-3 tablets po per meal or 5 drops per serving.[1]

Constipation predominant
- Bran or Psyllium 1 tbspn tid with meals; increase as needed
- Osmotic laxatives: Lactulose 1-2 tsp QHS PEG (polyethylene glycol) 8 oz QHS

Pain predominant

Post-prandial
- Dicliomine 10-20 mg 10-15 minutes prior to meals

↓

Referal to Pain Service

Chronic persistent
- Amitriptyline 25 mg QHS and increase as needed to maximum of 100 mg QHS
  OR
- Imipramine 25 mg QHS and increase as needed to maximum of 150 mg QHS

1. Effective in foods containing the sugars raffinose, stachyose, and/or verboscose found in oats, legumes and cruciferous vegetables.

60

5i: Clinical Approach to Acute Pancreatitis

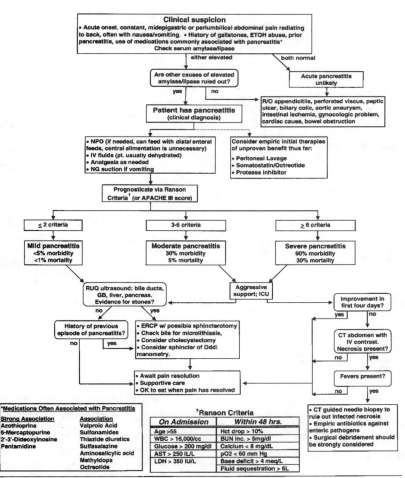

Clinical suspicion
- Acute onset, constant, midepigastric or periumbilical abdominal pain radiating to back, often with nausea/vomiting. • History of gallstones, ETOH abuse, prior pancreatitis, use of medications commonly associated with pancreatitis*
Check serum amylase/lipase

either elevated → **Are other causes of elevated amylase/lipase ruled out?**

both normal → **Acute pancreatitis unlikely**

yes / no

Patient has pancreatitis (clinical diagnosis)

R/O appendicitis, perforated viscus, peptic ulcer, biliary colic, aortic aneurysm, intestinal ischemia, gynocologic problem, cardiac cause, bowel obstruction

- NPO (if needed, can feed with *distal* enteral feeds, central alimentation is unnecessary)
- IV fluids (pt. usually dehydrated)
- Analgesia as needed
- NG suction if vomiting

Consider empiric initial therapies of unproven benefit thus far:
- Peritoneal Lavage
- Somatostatin/Octreotide
- Protease inhibitor

Prognosticate via Ranson Criteria[†] (or APACHE III score)

≤ 2 criteria → **Mild pancreatitis** <5% morbidity <1% mortality

3-5 criteria → **Moderate pancreatitis** 30% morbidity 5% mortality

≥ 6 criteria → **Severe pancreatitis** 90% morbidity 30% mortality

Aggressive support; ICU

RUQ ultrasound: bile ducts, GB, liver, pancreas. Evidence for stones?

no / yes

History of previous episode of pancreatitis?
no / yes

- ERCP w/ possible sphincterotomy
- Check bile for microlithiasis,
- Consider cholecystectomy
- Consider sphincter of Oddi manometry

- Await pain resolution
- Supportive care
- OK to eat when pain has resolved

Improvement in first four days?
yes / no

CT abdomen with IV contrast. Necrosis present?
no / yes

Fevers present?
no / yes

- CT guided needle biopsy to rule out infected necrosis
- Empiric antibiotics against enteric pathogens
- Surgical debridement should be strongly considered

---

*Medications Often Associated with Pancreatitis

Strong Association	Association
Azothioprine	Valproic Acid
6-Mercaptopurine	Sulfonamides
2'-3'-Dideoxyinosine	Thiazide diuretics
Pentamidine	Sulfasalazine
	Aminosalicylic acid
	Methyldopa
	Octreotide

[†]Ranson Criteria

On Admission	Within 48 hrs.
Age >55	Hct drop > 10%
WBC > 16,000/cc	BUN inc. > 5mg/dl
Glucose > 200 mg/dl	Calcium < 8 mg/dL
AST > 250 IL/L	pO2 < 60 mm Hg
LDH > 350 IU/L	Base deficit > 4 meq/L
	Fluid sequestration > 6L

1. Bank S, Indaram A. Causes of acute and recurrent pancreatitis. Clinical considerations and clues to diagnosis. Gastroenterol Clin North Am 1999 Sep;28(3):571-89
2. Munoz A, Katerndahi DA. Diagnosis and management of acute pancreatitis. Am Fam Phys 2000 Jul 1;62(1):164-74
3. Steinberg W Tenner S Acute pancreatitis NEJM 1994 330 (17):1198-210
4. Marshall JB Acute pancreatitis: A Review with an Emphasis on New Developments. Arch Int Med 1993 153(10):1185-98

5j: Acute Right Upper Quadrant Pain

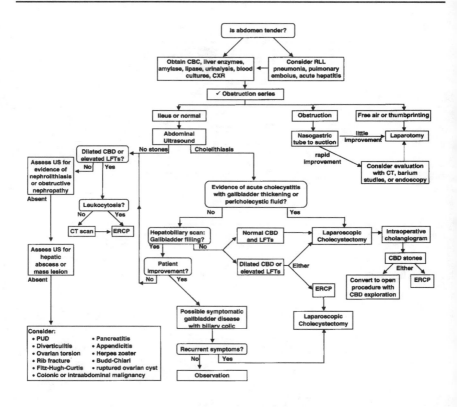

Abbreviations: US = ultrasound, CT = computed tomography, ERCP = endoscopic retrograde cholangiopancreatography, CBD = common bile duct, LFTs = liver function tests, PUD = peptic ulcer disease.

Erikson, RA and Carlson, B. The role of endoscopic retrograde cholangiopancreatography in patients with laparoscopic cholecystectomies. Gastroenterology 1995;109:252.

Rathgaber S. Right upper quadrant abdominal pain: Diagnosis in patients without evident gallstones. Postgraduate Med 1993;94:153

Paterson-Brown S, Vipond MN. Modern aids to clinical decision making in the acute abdomen. Br. J. Surg. 1990;77:13.

Brewer RJ, Golden GR, Hitch DC, et al. Abdominal pain: An analysis of 1000 consecutive cases in a university hospital emergency room. Am. J. Surg. 1976;131:219.

Bender JS. Approach to the acute abdomen. Med. Clin. N.A. 1989; 73:1413.

5k: Treatment of Inflammatory Bowel Disease - Crohn's Disease

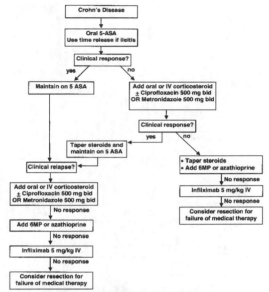

Agents Used in the Treatment of Inflammatory Bowel Disease

Category	Drug	Unit	Dose range	Site of Release
Oral 5-ASA	Sulfasalazine (Azulfidine)	500 mg	2-4 g/day: divided doses tid-qid	colon
Oral 5-ASA	Mesalamine (Asacol)	400 mg	2.4-4.8 g/day: divided doses tid-qid	colon/ileum
Oral 5-ASA	Mesalamine time release (Pentasa)	250 mg	3.0-4 g/day: divided doses tid-qid	duodenum to colon
Oral 5-ASA	Olsalazine (Dipentum)	250 mg	0.75 - 3.0 g/day: divided doses tid-qid	colon/ileum
5-ASA suppository	Mesalamine suppository	0.5 or 1 g	One suppository bid	rectum
5-ASA enema	Mesalamine enema	60 or 100 ml	4 g QD or bid	left colon
Oral corticosteroid	Oral steroid: prednisone*	5-20 mg	40-60 mg/day with subsequent taper	
IV corticosteroid	IV steroid: Hydrocortisone		100 mg Q 8H	
Corticosteroid enema	Hydrocortisone enema*	100 mg	100 mg QD or bid	left colon
Immunosuppressive†	6 mercaptopurine (6MP)	50 mg	1.0 - 1.5 mg/kg/day: single daily dose	
Immunosuppressive†	Azathioprine (Imuran)	50 mg	1.0-2.0 mg/kg/day: single daily dose	
Immunosuppressive†	IV cyclosporin		4 mg/kg/day	
Anti-TNFα†	IV Infliximab	5 mg/kg	Check product literature	

*Alternate day oral steroids have been shown to reduce side effects. Oral budesonide may have equal or greater efficacy with less systemic absorption (investigational)
† Immunosuppressive agents should be given only by physicians knowledgeable in their use (recommend subspecialist consultation)

5I: Treatment of Inflammatory Bowel Disease - Ulcerative Colitis

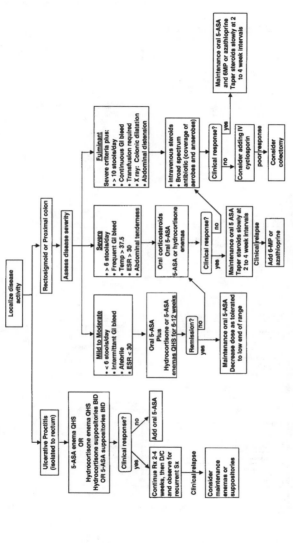

See *Agents used in the treatment of inflammatory bowel disease* in Crohn's disease algorithm for drug doses and abbreviations.

Baert FJ, Rutgeerts PJ. Medical Therapies for Ulcerative Colitis and Crohn's Disease. Curr Gastroenterol Rep 2(6):446-450, 2000

Elson CO. The basis of current and future therapy for inflammatory bowel disease. Am J Med 100:656- 662, 1996

Pearson DC, May GR, Fick GH, Sutherland LR. Azathioprine and 6 mercaptopurine in Crohn's disease, a meta-analysis. Ann Int Med 123:132-142, 1995

Hanauer SB. Inflammatory Bowel Disease. N Engl J Med 334:841-848, 1996

Sugar PM, Pemberton JH. Update on the surgical management of ulcerative colitis and ulcerative proctitis: current controversies and problems. Inflammatory Bowel Dis 1:299-312, 1996

5m: Elevated Liver Enzymes

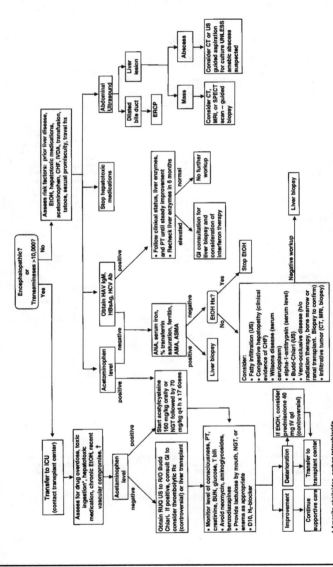

* Amanita phalloides, carbon tetrachloride
† Although viral antigens, viral antibodies, and ceruloplasmin should be obtained, they are not helpful in the acute setting. Liver biopsy in general is also not helpful in fulminant hepatic failure.

Abbreviations: EtOH = alcohol, CHF = congestive heart failure, IVDA = intravenous drug abuse, NGT = nasogastric tube, PT = prothrombin time, T Bili = total bilirubin, BUN = blood urea nitrogen, HAV = hepatitis A virus, HBsAg = hepatitis B virus surface antigen, HCV Ab= hepatitis C virus antibody, ANA = antinuclear antibody, AMA = antimitochondrial antibody, ASMA = anti-smooth muscle antibody, ERCP = endoscopic retrograde cholangiopancreatography, CT = computed tomography, MRI = magnetic resonance imaging, US = RUQ ultrasound, D₁₀ = 10% dextrose solution.

Pratt DS, Kaplan MM. Evaluation of abnormal liver-enzyme results in asymptomatic patients. N Engl J Med. 2000 Apr 27;342(17):1266-71
Herlong HF. Approach to the patient with abnormal liver enzymes. Hospital Practice 1994;29:32.
Lee, WM. Acute liver failure. NEJM 1993;329:1862.
Gitlin, NM. Therapeutic implications of the evaluation of liver enzymes. In: Current therapy in gastroenterology and liver disease (ed: T.M. Bayless) Mosby 1994 pg 474.

5n: Upper Gastrointestinal Bleeding

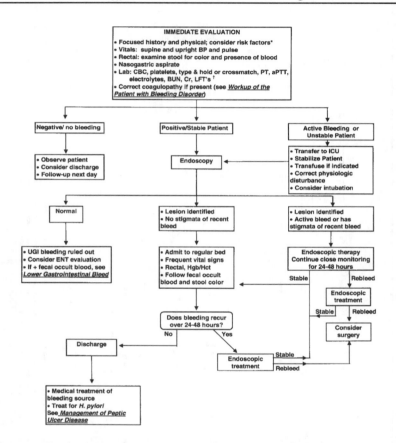

IMMEDIATE EVALUATION
- Focused history and physical; consider risk factors*
- Vitals: supine and upright BP and pulse
- Rectal: examine stool for color and presence of blood
- Nasogastric aspirate
- Lab: CBC, platelets, type & hold or crossmatch, PT, aPTT, electrolytes, BUN, Cr, LFT's †
- Correct coagulopathy if present (see *Workup of the Patient with Bleeding Disorder*)

Negative/ no bleeding
- Observe patient
- Consider discharge
- Follow-up next day

Positive/Stable Patient
→ Endoscopy

Active Bleeding or Unstable Patient
- Transfer to ICU
- Stabilize Patient
- Transfuse if indicated
- Correct physiologic disturbance
- Consider intubation

Normal
- UGI bleeding ruled out
- Consider ENT evaluation
- If + fecal occult blood, see *Lower Gastrointestinal Bleed*

- Lesion identified
- No stigmata of recent bleed

- Admit to regular bed
- Frequent vital signs
- Rectal, Hgb/Hct
- Follow fecal occult blood and stool color

- Lesion identified
- Active bleed or has stigmata of recent bleed

Endoscopic therapy Continue close monitoring for 24-48 hours

Stable | Rebleed

Endoscopic treatment

Stable | Rebleed

Consider surgery

Does bleeding recur over 24-48 hours?
No | Yes

Discharge

Endoscopic treatment
Stable | Rebleed

- Medical treatment of bleeding source
- Treat for *H. pylori*
See *Management of Peptic Ulcer Disease*

---

* Prompt initial exam should determine severity of situation. Focus history on likely cause of bleeding: liver disease, NSAIDS, alcohol, vomiting, ulcer, cancer, etc. Risk Factors: Morbidity, mortality and rebleed increase with these factors: current rebleed, large volume bleed, bleed while on treatment, recent ASA/NSAIDs, liver disease, CHF, CAD, renal failure, respiratory failure, hematologic malignancy and renal failure.

† Consider obtaining bleeding time, alcohol level, toxicology screen as appropriate. Consider ECG.

5o: Lower Gastrointestinal Bleeding

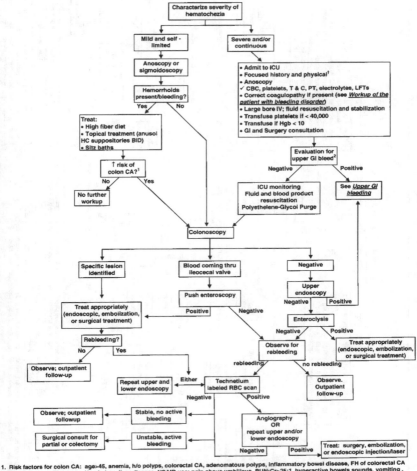

1. Risk factors for colon CA: age>45, anemia, h/o polyps, colorectal CA, adenomatous polyps, inflammatory bowel disease, FH of colorectal CA
2. Signs of upper GI source: Hx of ulcer, liver disease, NSAID use; pain above umbilicus, BUN:Cr>25:1, hyperactive bowels sounds, vomiting, positive nasogastric aspirate
LFTs – liver function tests. Enteroclysis – air contrast study.

6a: Acute Renal Failure

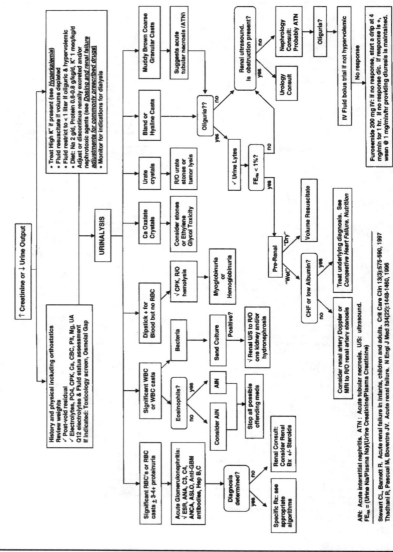

↑ Creatinine or ↓ Urine Output

History and physical including orthostatics
Review weights
√ Post-void residual
√ Electrolytes, PO4, CPK, Ca, CBC, Plt, Mg, UA
Q12 electrolytes & Fluid status assessment
If indicated: Toxicology screen, Osmolal Gap

• Treat High K+ if present (see *Hyperkalemia*)
• Fluid resuscitate if volume depleted
• Fluid restrict to < 1 liter if oliguric & hypervolemic
• Diet: Na 2 g/d, Protein 0.6–0.8 g/kg/d, K+ 1 meq/kg/d
  Adjust or discontinue renally excreted and/or
  nephrotoxic agents (see *Dosing and renal failure
  adjustments for commonly prescribed drugs*)
• Monitor for indications for dialysis

URINALYSIS

Significant RBC's or RBC casts ± 3-4+ proteinuria

Acute Glomerulonephritis:
√ ESR, ANA, C3, C4,
ANCA, ASLO, Anti-GBM
antibodies, Hep B,C

Diagnosis determined?
— yes → Specific Rx: see appropriate algorithms
— no → Renal Consult: Consider Renal Bx +/- Steroids

Significant WBC or WBC casts

Eosinophils?
— yes → AIN
— no → Consider AIN

Stop all possible offending meds

Bacteria → Send Culture → Positive? → √ Renal U/S to R/O one kidney and/or hydronephrosis

Dipstick + for Blood but no RBC

√ CPK, R/O hemolysis

Myoglobinuria or Hemoglobinuria

Ca Oxalate Crystals

Consider stones or Ethylene Glycol Toxicity

Urate crystals

R/O urate stones or tumor lysis

Bland or Hyaline Casts

Muddy Brown Coarse Granular Casts

Suggests acute tubular necrosis (ATN)

Oliguria??
— yes → √ Urine Lytes → FE_{Na} < 1%?
  — yes → Pre-Renal
    "Dry" → Volume Resuscitate
    "Wet" → CHF or low Albumin?
      — yes → Treat underlying diagnosis. See *Congestive Heart Failure, Nutrition*
      — no → Consider renal artery Doppler or MRI to R/O renal artery stenosis
  — no → Renal ultrasound. Is obstruction present?
— no → Oliguria?? → Renal ultrasound. Is obstruction present?

Renal ultrasound. Is obstruction present?
— yes → Urology Consult
— no → Nephrology Consult: Probably ATN

Oliguria?

IV Fluid bolus trial if not hypervolemic

No response

Furosemide 200 mg IV: If no response, start a drip at 4 mg/min for 1 hr. If no response is +, wean @ 1 mg/min/hr providing diuresis is maintained.

AIN: Acute interstitial nephritis. ATN : Acute tubular necrosis. U/S: ultrasound.
FE_{Na} = (Urine Na/Plasma Na)x(Urine Creatinine/Plasma Creatinine)

Stewart CL, Barnett R. Acute renal failure in infants, children and adults. Crit Care Clin 13(3):575-590, 1997
Thadhani R, Pascual M, Boventre JV. Acute renal failure. N Engl J Med 334(22):1448-1460, 1996

6b: Hypertension - Outpatient Therapy

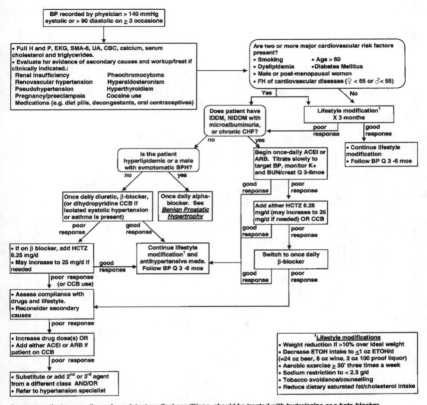

BP recorded by physician > 140 mmHg systolic or > 90 diastolic on ≥ 3 occasions

• Full H and P, EKG, SMA-6, UA, CBC, calcium, serum cholesterol and triglycerides.
• Evaluate for evidence of secondary causes and workup/treat if clinically indicated.:

Renal insufficiency	Pheochromocytoma
Renovascular hypertension	Hyperaldosteronism
Pseudohypertension	Hyperthyroidism
Pregnancy/preeclampsia	Cocaine use
Medications (e.g. diet pills, decongestants, oral contraceptives)	

Are two or more major cardiovascular risk factors present?
• Smoking   • Age > 60
• Dyslipidemia   •Diabetes Mellitus
• Male or post-menopausal woman
• FH of cardiovascular disease (♀ < 65 or ♂< 55)

Yes → Does patient have IDDM, NIDDM with microalbuminuria, or chronic CHF?

No → Lifestyle modification[1] X 3 months
- poor response → (down)
- good response → • Continue lifestyle modification • Follow BP Q 3 -6 mos

no → Is the patient hyperlipidemic or a male with symptomatic BPH?

yes (from Does patient have...) → Begin once-daily ACEI or ARB. Titrate slowly to target BP, monitor K+ and BUN/creat Q 3-6mos
- good response → Continue lifestyle modification[1] and antihypertensive meds. Follow BP Q 3 -6 mos
- poor response → Add either HCTZ 6.25 mg/d (may increase to 25 mg/d if needed) OR CCB
  - good response → Continue lifestyle modification...
  - poor response → Switch to once daily β-blocker
    - good response → Continue...
    - poor response → (down to Assess compliance)

no (hyperlipidemic) → Once daily diuretic, β-blocker, (or dihydropyridine CCB if isolated systolic hypertension or asthma is present)

yes → Once daily alpha-blocker. See *Benign Prostatic Hypertrophy*

- poor response (from Once daily diuretic...) → • If on β blocker, add HCTZ 6.25 mg/d • May increase to 25 mg/d if needed
- good response → Continue lifestyle modification[1] and antihypertensive meds. Follow BP Q 3 -6 mos
- good response → (Continue lifestyle modification)

poor response (or CCB use) → • Assess compliance with drugs and lifestyle. • Reconsider secondary causes

poor response → • Increase drug dose(s) OR • Add either ACEI or ARB if patient on CCB

poor response → • Substitute or add 2nd or 3rd agent from a different class AND/OR • Refer to hypertension specialist

[1]Lifestyle modifications
• Weight reduction if >10% over ideal weight
• Decrease ETOH intake to ≤1 oz ETOH/d (=24 oz beer, 8 oz wine, 2 oz 100 proof liquor)
• Aerobic exercise ≥ 30' three times a week
• Sodium restriction to < 2.3 g/d
• Tobacco avoidance/counselling
• Reduce dietary saturated fat/cholesterol intake

Pregnant patients, regardless of coexistent medical conditions, should be treated with hydralazine or a beta-blocker.
African Americans should be offered ACEI but are less likely than Caucasians to respond. A CCB may need to be substituted.

See *Dosing and renal failure adjustments for commonly prescribed drugs* for dosages of antihypertensive agents.
ACEI - Angiotensin converting enzyme inhibitor. ARB – angiotensin II receptor blocker. ACEIs and ARBs are contraindicated in pregnancy. BPH - Benign prostatic hyperplasia. CCB - calcium-channel blockers. FH – family history
HCTZ - hydrochlorthiazide

The Sixth Report of the Joint National Committee on Detection, Evaluation, and Treatment of High Blood Pressure. Arch Int Med 1997; 157:2413-46
Kaplan NM, Lieberman E. Clinical Hypertension. Baltimore, Williams & Wilkins; 180-192, 1990
Alderman MH. Which antihypertensive drugs first -- and why! JAMA 267: 2786 -2787, 1992

6c: Management of Acute Renal Colic

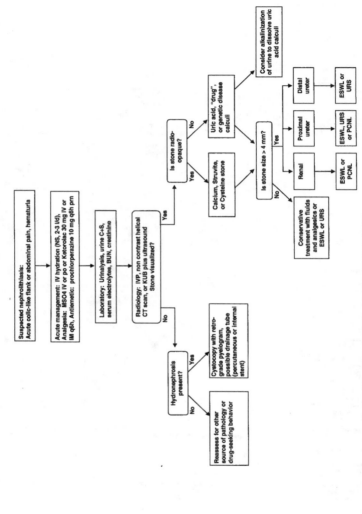

ESWL — extracorporeal shock wave lithotripsy, URS — ureteroscopy, PCNL — percutaneous nephrolithotomy

Saklayen MG. Medical management of nephrolithiasis. Med Clin NA 81: 785-799, 1997
Segura JW, Preminger GM, Assimos DG et al. Ureteral stones clinical guidelines panel summary report on the management of ureteral calculi. www.auanet.org/guidelines

6d: Metabolic Evaluation for Renal Calculi

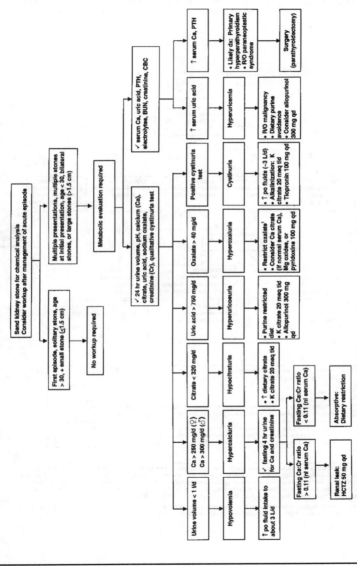

Send kidney stone for chemical analysis
Consider workup after management of acute episode

First episode, solitary stone, age > 30, + small stone (≤1.5 cm)
→ No workup required

Multiple presentations, multiple stones at initial presentation, age < 30, bilateral stones, or large stones (>1.5 cm)
→ Metabolic evaluation required

✓ 24 hr urine volume, pH, calcium (Ca), citrate, uric acid, sodium oxalate, creatinine (Cr), qualitative cystinuria test

Urine volume < 1 l/d	Ca > 250 mg/d (♀) Ca > 300 mg/d (♂)	Citrate < 320 mg/d	Uric acid > 750 mg/d	Oxalate > 40 mg/d	Positive cystinuria test
Hypovolemia	Hypercalciuria	Hypocitraturia	Hyperuricuria	Hyperoxaluria	Cystinuria

Hypovolemia
- ↑ po fluid intake to about 3 L/d

Hypercalciuria
✓ fasting 4 hr urine for Ca and creatinine

- Fasting Ca:Cr ratio > 0.11 (nl serum Ca) → Renal leak: HCTZ 50 mg qd
- Fasting Ca:Cr ratio < 0.11 (nl serum Ca) → Absorptive: Dietary restriction

Hypocitraturia
- ↑ dietary citrate
- K citrate 20 meq tid

Hyperuricuria
- Purine restricted diet
- K citrate 20 meq tid
- Allopurinol 300 mg qd

Hyperoxaluria
- Restrict oxalate[1]
- Consider Ca citrate (if normal serum Ca), Mg oxides, or pyridoxine 100 mg qd

Cystinuria
- ↑ po fluids (~3 L/d)
- Alkalinization: K citrate 20 meq tid
- Tiopronin 100 mg qd

✓ serum Ca, uric acid, PTH, electrolytes, BUN, creatinine, CBC

↑ serum uric acid	↑ serum Ca, PTH
Hyperuricemia	

Hyperuricemia
- R/O malignancy
- Dietary purine avoidance
- Consider allopurinol 300 mg qd

↑ serum Ca, PTH
- Likely dx: Primary hyperparathyroidism
- R/O paraneoplastic syndrome
→ Surgery (parathyroidectomy)

---

1. Foods which increase urinary oxalate: spinach, rhubarb, chocolate, peanuts, strawberry, tea, wheat bran, ascorbic acid

Saklayen MG. Medical management of nephrolithiasis. Med Clin NA 81: 785-799, 1997
Segura JW, Preminger GM, Assimos DG et al. Ureteral stones clinical guidelines panel summary report on the management of ureteral calculi. www.auanet.org/guidelines

71

6e: Workup of the Patient with Respiratory Acidosis

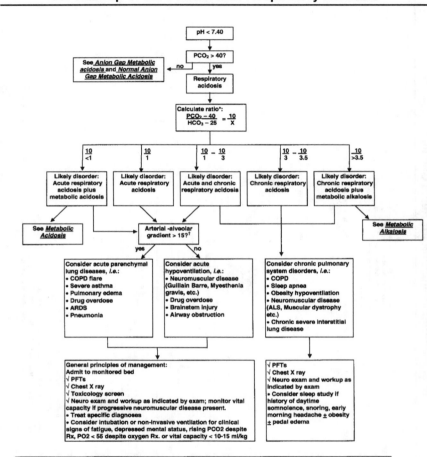

pH < 7.40

PCO₂ > 40?

See *Anion Gap Metabolic acidosis* and *Normal Anion Gap Metabolic Acidosis* ← no

yes

Respiratory acidosis

Calculate ratio*:
$$\frac{PCO_2 - 40}{HCO_3 - 25} = \frac{10}{X}$$

$\frac{10}{<1}$ $\frac{10}{1}$ $\frac{10}{1} - \frac{10}{3}$ $\frac{10}{3} - \frac{10}{3.5}$ $\frac{10}{>3.5}$

Likely disorder: Acute respiratory acidosis plus metabolic acidosis

Likely disorder: Acute respiratory acidosis

Likely disorder: Acute and chronic respiratory acidosis

Likely disorder: Chronic respiratory acidosis

Likely disorder: Chronic respiratory acidosis plus metabolic alkalosis

See *Metabolic Acidosis*

See *Metabolic Alkalosis*

Arterial-alveolar gradient > 15?[†]

yes   no

Consider acute parenchymal lung diseases, i.e.:
• COPD flare
• Severe asthma
• Pulmonary edema
• Drug overdose
• ARDS
• Pneumonia

Consider acute hypoventilation, i.e.:
• Neuromuscular disease (Guillian Barre, Myesthenia gravis, etc.)
• Drug overdose
• Brainstem injury
• Airway obstruction

Consider chronic pulmonary system disorders, i.e.:
• COPD
• Sleep apnea
• Obesity hypoventilation
• Neuromuscular disease (ALS, Muscular dystrophy etc.)
• Chronic severe interstitial lung disease

General principles of management:
Admit to monitored bed
√ PFTs
√ Chest X ray
√ Toxicology screen
√ Neuro exam and workup as indicated by exam; monitor vital capacity if progressive neuromuscular disease present.
• Treat specific diagnoses
• Consider intubation or non-invasive ventilation for clinical signs of fatigue, depressed mental status, rising PCO2 despite Rx, PO2 < 55 despite oxygen Rx. or vital capacity < 10-15 ml/kg

√ PFTs
√ Chest X ray
√ Neuro exam and workup as indicated by exam
• Consider sleep study if history of daytime somnolence, snoring, early morning headache ± obesity ± pedal edema

---

*These ratios can be estimated, but for some you will need a calculator. Examples: For a patient with a pCO2 of 45 and bicarb of 32, the ratio would be (45-40)/(32-25) = 5/7 ≈ 10/14, suggesting a respiratory acidosis with a metabolic alkalosis. A patient with a pCO2 of 53 and a bicarb of 20 would have a ratio of (53-40)/(20-25) = 13/-5 ≈ 10/-3.8. However, as the denominator is clearly < 1, the data easily can be seen to meet criteria for a concommittant metabolic acidosis without using a calculator.
[†] A-a gradient = PAO2 - PaO2 (from blood gas). PAO₂ =FIO₂((Pb-47) - PCO₂/R. Pb=barometric pressure.

Ratios within these ranges are consistent with, but not necessarily diagnostic of the disorders described. Complex acid-base disorders may mimic simple disorders. History and clinical correlation are required for interpretation.

6f: Anion Gap Metabolic Acidosis

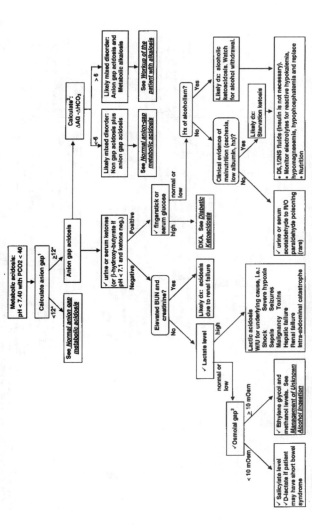

Complex acid-base disorders may mimic simple disorders. History and clinical correlation are required for interpretation.

1. Anion gap (AG): Na – (Cl+HCO3). The upper limit of normal will vary with the laboratory, check with your laboratory normals (varies from 10 to 15). The anion gap threshold is also lower if the albumin is < 4. If AG – [(12 – 2.5(4 – albumin)] is ≥ 2, then anion gap acidosis is present.

2. ΔAG = calculated anion gap – 12; ΔHCO3 = HCO3 – 24. Some authors use ≥ 8 or ≤ 4 as cutoff for a significant ΔAG– ΔHCO3 ("Δ- Δ"). We used a consensus mean of ± 6 in the above algorithm.
Δ-Δ within this range likely have a pure anion gap acidosis, Δ-Δ outside this range most commonly have the mixed disorders identified above.
• A simple way to do a similar calculation in your head: calculate anion gap, subtract 10, then add the serum bicarbonate. If the sum (= bicarb plus excess anion gap "bicarb equivalent") is ≥ 28, there is a concomittant metabolic alkalosis. If sum ≤ 20, there is a concomittant non-gap acidosis.

3. Osmolal gap: Measured osmolality – calculated osmolality. Calculated Osm = 2(Na) + Glucose/18 + BUN/2.8 + ethanol/4.6

Wrenn K. The delta gap: An approach to mixed acid base disorders. Ann Emerg Med 19: 1310-1313, 1990
Oster JR, Perez GO, Materson BJ. Use of the anion gap in clinical medicine. So Med J 81:229-237, 1988

6g: Normal Anion Gap Metabolic Acidosis

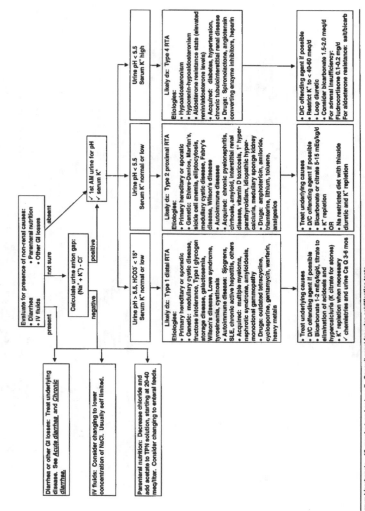

Evaluate for presence of non-renal causes:
- Diarrhea
- IV fluids
- Parenteral nutrition
- Other GI losses

present / not sure / absent

Calculate urine anion gap:
(Na⁺ + K⁺) - Cl⁻

negative / positive

✓ 1st AM urine for pH
✓ serum K⁺

Diarrhea or other GI losses: Treat underlying disease. See *Acute diarrhea* and *Chronic diarrhea*.

IV fluids: Consider changing to lower concentration of NaCl. Usually self limited.

Parenteral nutrition: Decrease chloride and add acetate to TPN solution, starting at 20-40 meq/liter. Consider changing to enteral feeds.

Urine pH > 5.5, HCO3 < 15*
Serum K⁺ normal or low

Likely dx: Type 1 distal RTA
Etiologies:
- Primary hereditary or sporadic
- Genetic: medullary cystic disease, fructose intolerance, Type I glycogen storage disease, galactosemia, Wilson's disease, Lowe syndrome, tyrosinemia, cystinosis
- Autoimmune diseases: Sjogrens, SLE, chronic active hepatitis, others
- Acquired: multiple myeloma, nephrotic syndrome, amyloidosis, monoclonal gammopathy
- Drugs: outdated tetracycline, cyclosporine, gentamycin, warfarin, heavy metals

- Treat underlying causes
- D/C offending agent if possible
- Bicarbonate 1-2 mEq/kg/d, titrate to elimination of acidosis and hypercalciuria (K citrate for stones)
- K⁺ repletion when necessary
- ✓ chemistries and urine Ca Q 3-6 mos

Urine pH < 5.5
Serum K⁺ normal or low

Likely dx: Type 2 proximal RTA
Etiologies:
- Primary hereditary or sporadic
- Genetic: Ehlers-Danlos, Marfan's, sickle cell anemia, elliptocytosis, medullary cystic disease, Fabry's disease, Wilson's disease
- Autoimmune diseases
- Acquired: chronic pyelonephritis, cirrhosis, amyloid, interstitial renal disease, vitamin D toxicosis, 1° hyperparathyroidism, idiopathic hypercalciuria, medullary sponge kidney
- Drugs: amphotericin, amiloride, triamterine, lithium, toluene, analgesics

- Treat underlying causes
- D/C offending agent if possible
- Bicarbonate or citrate 5-15 mEq/kg/d
- K⁺ repletion
  OR
- Na restricted diet with thiazide diuretic and K⁺ repletion

Urine pH < 5.5
Serum K⁺ high

Likely dx: Type 4 RTA
Etiologies:
- Hypoaldosteronism
- Hyporenin-hypoaldosteronism
- Aldosterone resistance state (elevated renin/aldosterone levels)
- Acquired: diabetes, hypertension, chronic tubulointerstitial renal disease
- Drugs: Spironolactone, angiotensin converting enzyme inhibitors, heparin

- D/C offending agent if possible
- Restrict K⁺ to < 40-60 meq/d
- Loop diuretic
- Consider bicarbonate 1.5-2.0 meq/d
For adrenal insufficiency:
Fludrocortisone 0.1-0.2 mg/d
For aldosterone resistance: salt/bicarb

---

* If serum bicarbonate > 15, may be type I or type II. Consult renal for urine acidification tests.
Smulders YM et al. Renal tubular acidosis: pathophysiology and diagnosis. Arch Intern Med 156: 1629-1636, 1996
Battle et al. The use of the urinary anion gap in the diagnosis of hyperchloremic metabolic acidosis. N Engl J Med 318: 594-599, 1988
Coe FL, Kathpalia S. Hereditary tubular disorders. In Wyngarden JB and Smith LH eds, Harrison's Principles of Internal Medicine, 13th ed, McGraw Hill, New York, 1326-1329, 1994

6h: Workup of the Patient with Alkalosis

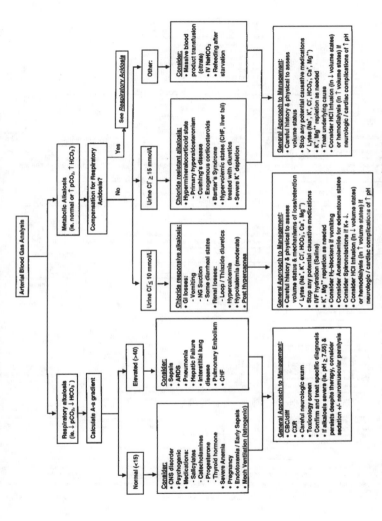

Arterial Blood Gas Analysis

Respiratory alkalosis (ie. ↓ pCO₂, ↓ HCO₃⁻)

Calculate A-a gradient

Normal (<15)

Consider:
- CNS disorder
- Psychogenic
- Medications:
  - Salicylates
  - Catecholamines
  - Progesterone
  - Thyroid hormone
- Severe Anemia
- Pregnancy
- Endotoxemia / Early Sepsis
- Mech Ventilation (iatrogenic)

Elevated (>40)

Consider:
- Sepsis
- ARDS
- Pneumonia
- Hepatic Failure
- Interstitial lung disease
- Pulmonary Embolism
- CHF

General Approach to Management:
- CBC/diff
- CXR
- Careful neurologic exam
- Toxicology screen
- Confirm and treat specific diagnosis
- If alkalosis severe (ie. pH ≥ 7.55) & persists despite therapy, consider sedation +/- neuromuscular paralysis

Metabolic Alkalosis (ie. normal or ↑ pCO₂, ↑ HCO₃⁻)

Compensation for Respiratory Acidosis?

Yes → See *Respiratory Acidosis*

No

Urine Cl⁻ ≤ 10 mmol/L

Chloride responsive alkalosis:
- GI losses:
  - Vomiting
  - NG Suction
  - Some diarrheal states
- Renal losses:
  - Loop / Thiazide diuretics
- Hypercalcemia
- Hypokalemia (moderate)
- Post Hypercapnea

General Approach to Management:
- Careful history & physical to assess volume status & mechanisms of loss/retention
- ✓ Lytes (Na⁺, K⁺, Cl⁻, HCO₃⁻, Ca⁺, Mg⁺)
- Stop any potential causative medications
- IVF hydration (Saline)
- K⁺, Mg⁺ repletion as needed
- Consider H₂-blockers if vomiting
- Consider Acetazolamide for edematous states
- Consider Spironolactone if K⁺ ↓
- Consider HCl Infusion (in ↓ voluma states) or hemodialysis (in ↑ volume states) if neurologic / cardiac complications of ↑ pH

Urine Cl⁻ ≥ 16 mmol/L

Chloride resistant alkalosis:
- Hypermineralocorticoid state:
  - Primary hyperaldosteronism
  - Cushing's disease
  - Exogenous corticosteroids
- Bartter's Syndrome
- Hypervolemic states (CHF, liver fail) treated with diuretics
- Severe K⁺ depletion

Other:

Consider:
- Massive blood product transfusion (citrate)
- IV NaHCO₃
- Refeeding after starvation

General Approach to Management:
- Careful history & physical to assess volume status
- Stop any potential causative medications
- ✓ Lytes (Na⁺, K⁺, Cl⁻, HCO₃⁻, Ca⁺, Mg⁺)
- K⁺, Mg⁺ repletion as needed
- Treat underlying cause
- Consider HCl infusion (in ↓ volume states) or hemodialysis (in ↑ volume states) if neurologic / cardiac complications of ↑ pH

1. Black, RM Metabolic Acidosis and Metabolic Alkalosis. In *Intensive Care Medicine*: Rippe, Irwin, Fink, Cerra (eds) 3rd ed. Little Brown & Co. Boston, 1996. Chapter 80, pp 993 - 998.
2. Don, H Metabolic Alkalosis. In *Decision Making in Critical Care*: Don (ed.) BC Decker, Inc. Philadelphia, 1985. Pages 166 - 167.

7a: Hyponatremia

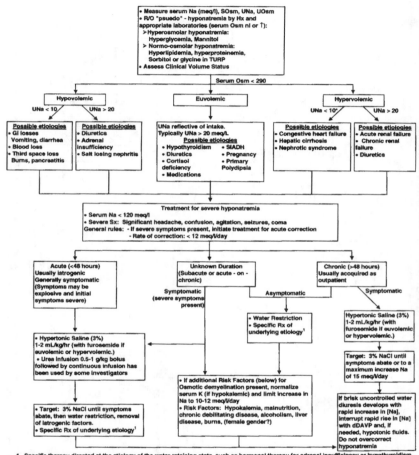

- Measure serum Na (meq/l), SOsm, UNa, UOsm
- R/O "psuedo" - hyponatremia by Hx and appropriate laboratories (serum Osm nl or ↑):
  - ➤ Hyperosmolar hyponatremia:
    Hyperglycemia, Mannitol
  - ➤ Normo-osmolar hyponatremia:
    Hyperlipidemia, hyperproteinemia,
    Sorbitol or glycine in TURP
- Assess Clinical Volume Status

Serum Osm < 290

Hypovolemic

UNa < 10 | UNa > 20

Possible etiologies
- GI losses
  Vomiting, diarrhea
- Blood loss
- Third space loss
  Burns, pancreatitis

Possible etiologies
- Diuretics
- Adrenal insufficiency
- Salt losing nephritis

Euvolemic

UNa reflective of intake.
Typically UNa > 20 meq/L
Possible etiologies
- Hypothyroidism
- Diuretics
- Cortisol deficiency
- Medications
- SIADH
- Pregnancy
- Primary Polydipsia

Hypervolemic

UNa < 10* | UNa > 20

Possible etiologies
- Congestive heart failure
- Hepatic cirrhosis
- Nephrotic syndrome

Possible etiologies
- Acute renal failure
- Chronic renal failure
- Diuretics

Treatment for severe hyponatremia
- Serum Na < 120 meq/l
- Severe Sx: Significant headache, confusion, agitation, seizures, coma
General rules: - If severe symptoms present, initiate treatment for acute correction
             - Rate of correction: < 12 meq/l/day

Acute (<48 hours)
Usually iatrogenic
Generally symptomatic
(Symptoms may be explosive and initial symptoms severe)

- Hypertonic Saline (3%)
  1-2 mL/kg/hr (with furosemide if euvolemic or hypervolemic.)
- Urea infusion 0.5-1 g/kg bolus followed by continuous infusion has been used by some investigators

- Target: 3% NaCl until symptoms abate, then water restriction, removal of iatrogenic factors.
- Specific Rx of underlying etiology[1]

Unknown Duration
(Subacute or acute - on - chronic)

Symptomatic
(severe symptoms present)

Asymptomatic

- Water Restriction
- Specific Rx of underlying etiology[1]

- If additional Risk Factors (below) for Osmotic demyelination present, normalize serum K (if hypokalemic) and limit increase in Na to 10-12 meq/l/day
- Risk Factors: Hypokalemia, malnutrition, chronic debilitating disease, alcoholism, liver disease, burns, (female gender?)

Chronic (>48 hours)
Usually acquired as outpatient

Symptomatic

Hypertonic Saline (3%) 1-2 mL/kg/hr (with furosemide if euvolemic or hypervolemic.)

Target: 3% NaCl until symptoms abate or to a maximum increase Na of 15 meq/l/day

If brisk uncontrolled water diuresis develops with rapid increase in [Na], interrupt rapid rise in [Na] with dDAVP and, if needed, hypotonic fluids. Do not overcorrect hyponatremia

1. Specific therapy directed at the etiology of the water retaining state, such as hormonal therapy for adrenal insufficiency or hypothyroidism, discontinuation of thiazide diuretics or other implicated medications, isotonic volume repletion in volume depleted states.

Berl T, Schreier RW. Disorders of water metabolism. In Schrier editor: Renal and Electrolyte Disorders 4th edition, Boston, Toronto and London, Little Brown and Company 1992
Soupart A, Decaux G. Therapeutic recommendations for management of severe hyponatremia. Clinical Nephrology 46: 149-169, 1996

7b: Hypernatremia

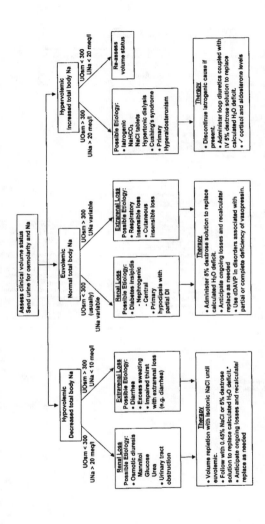

Assess clinical volume status
Send urine for osmolarity and Na

Hypovolemic
Decreased total body Na

UOsm > 300
UNa > 20 meq/l

Renal Loss
Possible Etiology:
- Osmotic diuresis
  - Mannitol
  - Glucose
  - Urea
- Urinary tract obstruction

UOsm > 300
UNa < 10 meq/l

Extrarenal Loss
Possible Etiology:
- Diarrhea
- Excess sweating
- Impaired thirst with extrarenal loss (e.g. diarrhea)

Therapy
- Volume repletion with isotonic NaCl until euvolemic.
- Follow with 0.45% NaCl or 5% dextrose solution to replace calculated H₂O deficit.*
- Anticipate ongoing losses and recalculate/ replace as needed

Euvolemic
Normal total body Na

UOsm > 300
(usually)
UNa variable

Renal Loss
Possible Etiology:
- Diabetes insipidis
  - Nephrogenic
  - Central
- Primary hypodipsia with partial DI

UOsm > 300
UNa variable

Extrarenal Loss
Possible Etiology:
- Respiratory insensible loss
- Cutaneous insensible loss

Therapy
- Administer 5% dextrose solution to replace calculated H₂O deficit.
- Anticipate ongoing losses and recalculate/ replace as needed
- Use dDAVP in disorders associated with partial or complete deficiency of vasopressin.

Hypervolemic
Increased total body Na

UOsm > 300
UNa > 20 meq/l

Possible Etiology:
- Iatrogenic
  - NaHCO₃
  - NaCl tablets
  - Hypertonic dialysis
- Cushing's syndrome
- Primary Hyperaldosteronism

UOsm < 300
UNa < 20 meq/l

Re-assess volume status

Therapy
- Discontinue iatrogenic cause if present.
- Administer loop diuretics coupled with iv 5% dextrose solution to replace calculated H₂O deficit.
- ✓ cortisol and aldosterone levels

Rate of Correction
- Water deficit should be corrected *gradually*, over more than 48 hours.
- The rate of decrease in serum Na should not exceed 1 meq/hr
- The drop in Osmolality should not exceed 2 mOsm/hr
- More rapid correction is associated with seizures, thought to be secondary to acute cerebral edema.

---

*Calculation of H₂O deficit

Observed Total body H₂O = Observed Weight (kg) X 0.6

$$Desired\ Total\ Body\ H_2O = \frac{Observed\ Na}{Target\ Na} \times Observed\ Total\ body\ H_2O$$

H₂O deficit = Desired Total Body H₂O - Observed Total body H₂O

Example: Observed Total body H₂O = 60kg X 0.6 = 36 L

$$Desired\ Total\ Body\ H_2O = \frac{165}{140} \times 36\ L = 42.4\ L.$$

H₂O deficit = 42.4 L - 36 L = 6.4 L

Beri T, Schrier RW. Disorders of water metabolism. In Schrier editor: Renal and Electrolyte Disorders 4th edition, Boston, Toronto and London, Little Brown and Company 1992
Sterns RH, Spital A. Disorders of water balance. In Kokko, Tannen editors: Fluid and Electrolytes, Philadelphia, WB Saunders, 1990.

7c: Hypokalemia

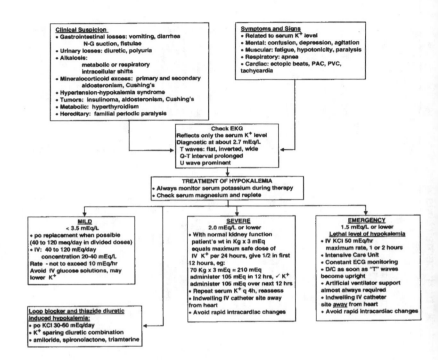

Clinical Suspicion
- Gastrointestinal losses: vomiting, diarrhea
  N-G suction, fistulae
- Urinary losses: diuretic, polyuria
- Alkalosis:
  metabolic or respiratory
  intracellular shifts
- Mineralocorticoid excess: primary and secondary
  aldosteronism, Cushing's
- Hypertension-hypokalemia syndrome
- Tumors: insulinoma, aldosteronism, Cushing's
- Metabolic: hyperthyroidism
- Hereditary: familial periodic paralysis

Symptoms and Signs
- Related to serum K^+ level
- Mental: confusion, depression, agitation
- Muscular: fatigue, hypotonicity, paralysis
- Respiratory: apnea
- Cardiac: ectopic beats, PAC, PVC,
  tachycardia

Check EKG
Reflects only the serum K^+ level
Diagnostic at about 2.7 mEq/L
T waves: flat, inverted, wide
Q-T interval prolonged
U wave prominent

TREATMENT OF HYPOKALEMIA
- Always monitor serum potassium during therapy
- Check serum magnesium and replete

MILD
< 3.5 mEq/L
- po replacement when possible
  (40 to 120 meq/day in divided doses)
- IV: 40 to 120 mEq/day
  concentration 20-40 mEq/L
  Rate - not to exceed 10 mEq/hr
  Avoid IV glucose solutions, may
  lower K^+

SEVERE
2.0 mEq/L or lower
- With normal kidney function
  patient's wt in Kg x 3 mEq
  equals maximum safe dose of
  IV K^+ per 24 hours, give 1/2 in first
  12 hours, eg:
  70 Kg x 3 mEq = 210 mEq
  administer 105 mEq in 12 hrs, ✓ K^+
  administer 105 mEq over next 12 hrs
- Repeat serum K^+ q 4h, reassess
- Indwelling IV catheter site away
  from heart
- Avoid rapid intracardiac changes

EMERGENCY
1.5 mEq/L or lower
Lethal level of hypokalemia
- IV KCl 50 mEq/hr
  maximum rate, 1 or 2 hours
- Intensive Care Unit
- Constant ECG monitoring
- D/C as soon as "T" waves
  become upright
- Artificial ventilator support
  almost always required
- Indwelling IV catheter
  site away from heart
- Avoid rapid intracardiac changes

**Loop blocker and thiazide diuretic
induced hypokalemia:**
- po KCl 30-60 mEq/day
- K^+ sparing diuretic combination
- amiloride, spironolactone, triamterine

Most cases require potassium replacement as KCl especially if alkalosis co-exists
In cases of metabolic acidosis, consider using K acetate, gluconate, or citrate (bicarbonate precursors)

7d: Hyperkalemia

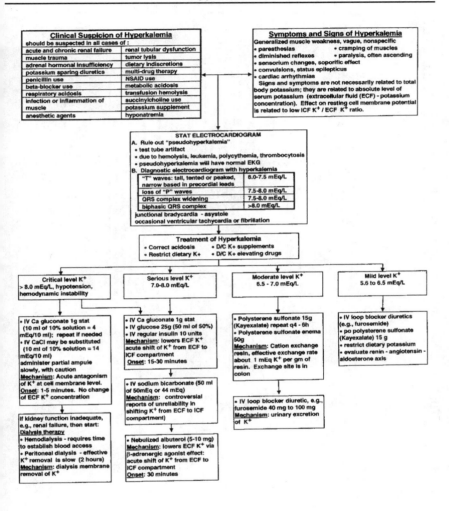

Clinical Suspicion of Hyperkalemia
should be suspected in all cases of :

acute and chronic renal failure	renal tubular dysfunction
muscle trauma	tumor lysis
adrenal hormonal insufficiency	dietary indiscretions
potassium sparing diuretics	multi-drug therapy
penicillin use	NSAID use
beta-blocker use	metabolic acidosis
respiratory acidosis	transfusion hemolysis
infection or inflammation of	succinylcholine use
muscle	potassium supplement
anesthetic agents	hyponatremia

Symptoms and Signs of Hyperkalemia
Generalized muscle weakness, vague, nonspecific
- paresthesias • cramping of muscles
- diminished reflexes • paralysis, often ascending
- sensorium changes, soporific effect
- convulsions, status epilepticus
- cardiac arrhythmias

Signs and symptoms are not necessarily related to total body potassium; they are related to absolute level of serum potassium (extracellular fluid (ECF) - potassium concentration). Effect on resting cell membrane potential is related to low ICF K^+ / ECF K^+ ratio.

STAT ELECTROCARDIOGRAM
A. Rule out "pseudohyperkalemia"
- test tube artifact
- due to hemolysis, leukemia, polycythemia, thrombocytosis
- pseudohyperkalemia will have normal EKG
B. Diagnostic electrocardiogram with hyperkalemia

"T" waves: tall, tented or peaked, narrow based in precordial leads	6.0-7.5 mEq/L
loss of "P" waves	7.5-8.0 mEq/L
QRS complex widening	7.5-8.0 mEq/L
biphasic QRS complex	>8.0 mEq/L

junctional bradycardia - asystole
occasional ventricular tachycardia or fibrillation

Treatment of Hyperkalemia
- Correct acidosis • D/C K+ supplements
- Restrict dietary K+ • D/C K+ elevating drugs

Critical level K^+
> 8.0 mEq/L, hypotension, hemodynamic instability

- IV Ca gluconate 1g stat (10 ml of 10% solution = 4 mEq/10 ml); repeat if needed
- IV CaCl may be substituted (10 ml of 10% solution = 14 mEq/10 ml) administer partial ampule slowly, with caution
Mechanism: Acute antagonism of K^+ at cell membrane level.
Onset: 1-5 minutes. No change of ECF K^+ concentration

If kidney function inadequate, e.g., renal failure, then start:
Dialysis therapy
- Hemodialysis - requires time to establish blood access
- Peritoneal dialysis - effective K^+ removal is slow (2 hours)
Mechanism: dialysis membrane removal of K^+

Serious level K^+
7.0-8.0 mEq/L

- IV Ca gluconate 1g stat
- IV glucose 25g (50 ml of 50%)
- IV regular insulin 10 units
Mechanism: lowers ECF K^+ acute shift of K^+ from ECF to ICF compartment
Onset: 15-30 minutes

- IV sodium bicarbonate (50 ml of 50mEq or 44 mEq)
Mechanism: controversial reports of unreliability in shifting K^+ from ECF to ICF compartment

- Nebulized albuterol (5-10 mg)
Mechanism: lowers ECF K^+ via β-adrenergic agonist effect: acute shift of K^+ from ECF to ICF compartment
Onset: 30 minutes

Moderate level K^+
6.5 - 7.0 mEq/L

- Polysterene sulfonate 15g (Kayexalate) repeat q4 - 6h
- Polysterene sulfonate enema 50g
Mechanism: Cation exchange resin, effective exchange rate about 1 mEq K^+ per gm of resin. Exchange site is in colon

- IV loop blocker diuretic, e.g., furosemide 40 mg to 100 mg
Mechanism: urinary excretion of K^+

Mild level K^+
5.5 to 6.5 mEq/L

- IV loop blocker diuretics (e.g., furosemide)
- po polysterene sulfonate (Kayexalate) 15 g
- restrict dietary potassium
- evaluate renin - angiotensin - aldosterone axis

7e: Evaluation and Management of Hypocalcemia

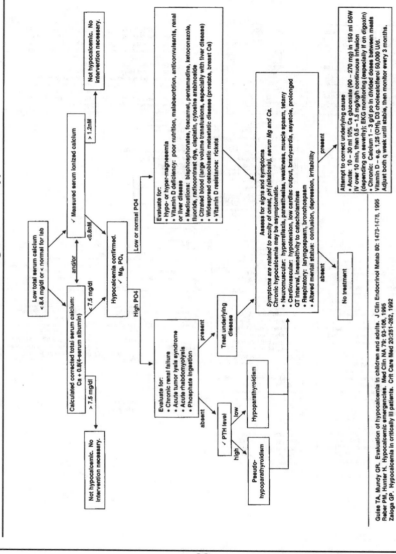

Low total serum calcium < 8.4 mg/dl or < normal for lab

Not hypocalcemic. No intervention necessary.

and/or

Measured serum ionized calcium

Calculated corrected total serum calcium: Ca + 0.8(4-serum albumin)

> 7.5 mg/dl — Not hypocalcemic. No intervention necessary.

< 7.5 mg/dl

< 0.8mM

> 1.2mM — Not hypocalcemic. No intervention necessary.

Hypocalcemia confirmed. ✓ Mg, PO₄

Low or normal PO4

High PO4

Evaluate for:
• Chronic renal failure
• Acute tumor lysis syndrome
• Acute rhabdomyolysis
• Phosphate ingestion

present — Treat underlying disease

absent

✓ PTH level

low — Hypoparathyroidism

high — Pseudo-hypoparathyroidism

Evaluate for:
• Hypo- or hyper-magnesemia
• Vitamin D deficiency: poor nutrition, malabsorption, anticonvulsants, renal or liver disease
• Medications: bisphosphonates, foscarnet, pentamadine, ketoconazole, fluoride, radiocontrast dye, cisplatin, cytosine arabinoside
• Citrated blood (large volume transfusions, especially with liver disease)
• Widespread osteoblastic metastatic disease (prostate, breast Ca)
• Vitamin D resistance: rickets

Assess for signs and symptoms

Symptoms are related to acuity of onset, pH (alkalosis), serum Mg and Ca.
Chronic hypocalcemia may be asymptomatic.
• Neuromuscular: hyperreflexia, paresthesias, weakness, muscle spasm, tetany
• Cardiovascular: hypotension, low cardiac output, bradycardia, asystole, prolonged QT interval, insensitivity to catecholamines
• Respiratory: laryngospasm, bronchospasm
• Altered mental status: confusion, depression, irritability

present

Attempt to correct underlying cause
• Acute: 10 – 30 ml 10% Ca gluconate (90 – 270 mg) in 150 ml D5W IV over 10 min, then 0.5 – 1.5 mg/kg/h continuous infusion (depending on severity); EKG monitoring (especially if on digoxin)
• Chronic: Calcium 1 – 3 g/d po in divided doses between meals
  Vitamin D – e.g. 1,25 (OH)₂ D3 cholecalciferol 50,000 U/d.
  Adjust both q week until stable, then monitor every 3 months.

absent — No treatment

Guise TA, Mundy GR. Evaluation of hypocalcemia in children and adults. J Clin Endocrinol Metab 80: 1473-1478, 1995
Reber PM, Hunter H. Hypocalcemic emergencies. Med Clin NA 79: 93-106, 1995
Zaloga GP. Hypocalcemia in critically ill patients. Crit Care Med 20:251-262, 1992

7f: Evaluation and Management of Hypercalcemia

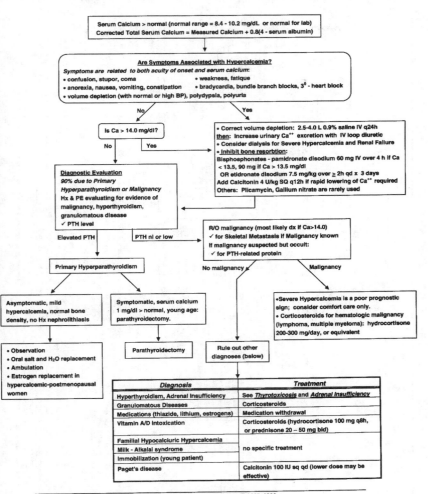

Serum Calcium > normal (normal range = 8.4 - 10.2 mg/dL or normal for lab)
Corrected Total Serum Calcium = Measured Calcium + 0.8(4 - serum albumin)

Are Symptoms Associated with Hypercalcemia?
Symptoms are related to both acuity of onset and serum calcium:
- confusion, stupor, coma
- anorexia, nausea, vomiting, constipation
- volume depletion (with normal or high BP), polydypsia, polyuria
- weakness, fatigue
- bradycardia, bundle branch blocks, 3° - heart block

No / Yes

Is Ca > 14.0 mg/dl?

No / Yes

- Correct volume depletion: 2.5-4.0 L 0.9% saline IV q24h
  then: increase urinary Ca^{++} excretion with IV loop diuretic
- Consider dialysis for Severe Hypercalcemia and Renal Failure
- Inhibit bone resorbtion:
  Bisphosphonates - pamidronate disodium 60 mg IV over 4 h if Ca < 13.5, 90 mg if Ca > 13.5 mg/dl
  OR etidronate disodium 7.5 mg/kg over ≥ 2h qd x 3 days
  Add Calcitonin 4 U/kg SQ q12h if rapid lowering of Ca^{++} required
  Others: Plicamycin, Gallium nitrate are rarely used

Diagnostic Evaluation
*90% due to Primary
Hyperparathyroidism or Malignancy*
Hx & PE evaluating for evidence of
malignancy, hyperthyroidism,
granulomatous disease
✓ PTH level

Elevated PTH / PTH nl or low

R/O malignancy (most likely dx if Ca>14.0)
✓ for Skeletal Metastasis if Malignancy known
If malignancy suspected but occult:
✓ for PTH-related protein

No malignancy / Malignancy

Primary Hyperparathyroidism

Asymptomatic, mild
hypercalcemia, normal bone
density, no Hx nephrolithiasis

Symptomatic, serum calcium
1 mg/dl > normal, young age:
parathyroidectomy.

- •Severe Hypercalcemia is a poor prognostic
  sign; consider comfort care only.
- Corticosteroids for hematologic malignancy
  (lymphoma, multiple myeloma): hydrocortisone
  200-300 mg/day, or equivalent

- Observation
- Oral salt and H_2O replacement
- Ambulation
- Estrogen replacement in
  hypercalcemic-postmenopausal
  women

Parathyroidectomy

Rule out other
diagnoses (below)

Diagnosis	Treatment
Hyperthyroidism, Adrenal Insufficiency	See *Thyrotoxicosis* and *Adrenal Insufficiency*
Granulomatous Diseases	Corticosteroids
Medications (thiazide, lithium, estrogens)	Medication withdrawal
Vitamin A/D intoxication	Corticosteroids (hydrocortisone 100 mg q8h, or prednisone 20 – 50 mg bid)
Familial Hypocalciuric Hypercalcemia	
Milk - Alkalai syndrome	no specific treatment
Immobilization (young patient)	
Paget's disease	Calcitonin 100 IU sq qd (lower dose may be effective)

Bilezikian JP. Management of Hypercalcemia. J Clin Endocrinol Metab 77:1445, 1993.
Edelson GW, Kleerekoper M. Hypercalcemic Crisis Med Clin North Am 79:79, 1995.

8a: Urinary Tract Infections

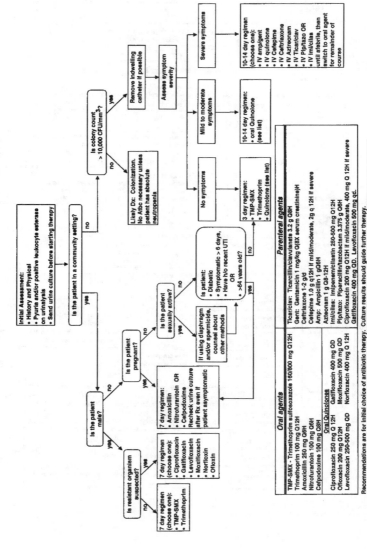

Initial Assessment:
- History and Physical
- Pyuria and/or positive leukocyte esterase on urinalysis
- Send urine culture before starting therapy

Is the patient in a community setting?

Is the patient male?

Is resistant organism suspected?

7 day regimen (choose one):
- TMP-SMX
- Trimethoprim

7 day regimen (choose one):
- Ciprofloxacin
- Gatifloxacin
- Levofloxacin
- Moxifloxacin
- Norfloxacin
- Ofloxin

Is the patient pregnant?

7 day regimen:
- Amoxicillin
- Nitrofurantoin OR
- Cefpodoxime

Recheck urine culture after Rx even if patient asymptomatic

Is the patient sexually active?

If using diaphragm and/or spermicide, counsel about other methods

Is patient:
- Diabetic
- Symptomatic > 6 days, OR
- Have h/o recent UTI
OR
- >64 years old?

3 day regimen:
- TMP-SMX
- Trimethoprim
- Quinolone (see list)

Is colony count > 10,000 CFU/mm³?

Likely Dx: Colonization. No Atbc necessary unless patient has absolute neutropenia

Remove indwelling catheter if possible

Assess symptom severity

No symptoms

Mild to moderate symptoms

Severe symptoms

10-14 day regimen:
- oral Quinolone (see list)

10-14 day regimen (choose one):
- IV ampi/gent
- IV quinolone
- IV Cefepime
- IV Ceftriaxone
- IV Aztreonam
- IV Ticar/clav
- IV Pip/tazo OR
- IV Imi/cilas
until afebrile, then switch to oral agent for remainder of course

---

Oral agents

TMP-SMX - Trimethoprim sulfoexazole 160/800 mg Q12H
Trimethoprim 100 mg Q12H
Amoxicillin 250 mg Q8H
Nitrofurantoin 100 mg Q6H
Cefpodoxime 100 mg Q8H

Oral Quinolones
Ciprofloxacin 250 mg Q 12H
Ofloxacin 500 mg QD
Levofloxacin 250-500 mg Q 12H

Gatifloxacin 400 mg QD
Moxifloxacin 400 mg QD
Norfloxacin 400 mg Q 12H

Parenteral agents

Ticar/clav: Ticarcillin/clavulanate 3.2 g Q8H
Gent: Gentamicin 1 mg/kg Q(8X serum creatinine)H
Ceftriaxone 1-2 g/d
Cefepime 1.0 g Q12H if mild/moderate, 2g q 12H if severe
Amp: Ampicillin 1 gQ6H
Aztreonam 1 g Q8-12H
Imi/cilas: Imipenem/cilastin 250-500 mg Q12H
Pip/tazo: Piperacillin/tazobactam 3.375 g Q6H
Ciprofloxacin 200 mg Q12H if mild/moderate, 400 mg Q 12H if severe
Gatifloxacin 400 mg QD, Levofloxacin 500 mg qd.

Recommendations are for initial choice of antibiotic therapy. Culture results should guide further therapy.

Stamm WE, Hooten TM. Management of urinary tract infections in adults. N Engl J Med 329: 1328-34, 1993
Neu HC. Urinary tract infections. Am J Med 92 (4A):63S-70S, 1992
Wilkie ME, Almond MK, Marsh FP. Diagnosis and management of urinary tract infections in adults. BMJ 305:1137-1141, 1992

8b: Vaginitis

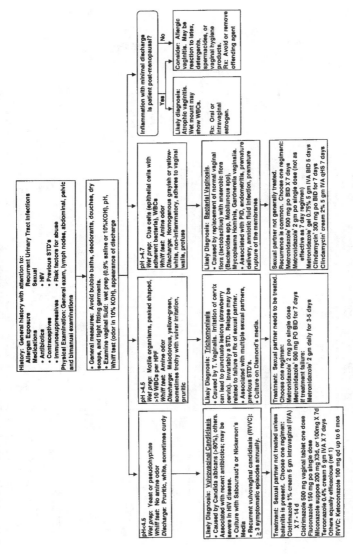

History: General history with attention to:
- Allergen Exposure
- Medications
  - Antibiotics
  - Contraceptives
  - Immunosuppressives

- Recurrent Urinary Tract Infections
- Sexual
  - HIV
  - Previous STD's
  - Risk factors for abuse

Physical Examination: General exam, lymph nodes, abdominal, pelvic and bimanual examinations

- General measures: Avoid bubble baths, deodorants, douches, dry soaps, and tight fitting garments.
- Examine vaginal fluid: wet prep (0.9% saline or 10%KOH), pH, Whiff test (odor in 10% KOH), appearance of discharge

---

pH<4.5
Wet prep: Yeast or pseudohyphae
Whiff test: No amine odor
Discharge: Pruritic, white, sometimes curdy

Likely Diagnosis: Vulvovaginal Candidiasis:
- Caused by Candida albicans (>90%), others. Associated with recent antibiotics; may be severe in HIV disease.
- Culture with Sabouraud's or Nickerson's Media
- Recurrent vulvovaginal candidiasis (RVVC): ≥ 3 symptomatic episodes annually.

Treatment: Sexual partner not treated unless balanitis is present. Choose one regimen:
Clotrimazole 1% cream 5 gm Intravaginal (IVA) X 7 - 14 d
Clotrimazole 500 mg vaginal tablet one dose
Fluconazole 150 mg po single dose
Miconazole suppo 200 mg 3/3d, or 100mg X 7d
Terconazole 0.4% cream 5 gm IVA X 7 days
Others equally efficacious (ref 1)
RVVC: Ketoconazole 100 mg qd up to 6 mos

---

pH >4.5
Wet prep: Motile organisms, peaked shaped, >10 WBCs per HPF
Whiff test: Amine odor
Discharge: Malodorous, yellow-green, sometimes frothy with vulvar irritation, pruritic.

Likely Diagnosis: Trichomoniasis
- Caused by T. Vaginalis. Irritation of cervix can lead to punctate lesions (strawberry cervix). Invariably a STD. Relapse may be related to failure of Rx of sexual partner.
- Associated with multiple sexual partners, previous STD's.
- Culture on Diamond's media.

Treatment: Sexual partner needs to be treated. Choose one regimen:
Metronidazole[1] 2 gm po single dose
Metronidazole[1] 500 mg BID for 7 days
If treatment failure:
Metronidazole[1] 2 gm daily for 3-5 days

---

pH >4.7
Wet prep: Clue cells (epithelial cells with adherent bacteria), WBCs
Whiff test: Amine odor
Discharge: Homogenous grayish or yellow-white, non-inflammatory, adhere to vaginal walls, profuse

Likely Diagnosis: Bacterial Vaginosis:
- Caused by replacement of normal vaginal flora (lactobacillus) with anaerobic flora (Bacteroides spp, Mobiluncus spp), Mycoplasma hominis, Gardnerella vaginalis.
- Associated with PID, endometritis, premature delivery, amniotic fluid infection, premature rupture of the membranes

Sexual partner not generally treated. Recurrence is common. Choose one regimen:
Metronidazole[1] 500 mg po BID X 7 days
Metronidazole[1] 2 gm po single dose (not as effective as 7 day regimen)
Metronidazole[1] gel 0.75% 5 gm IVA BID 5 days
Clindamycin[1] 300 mg po BID for 7 days
Clindamycin[1] cream 2% 5 gm IVA qhS 7 days

Inflammation with minimal discharge is patient post-menopausal?

Yes
Likely diagnosis: Atrophic Vaginitis. Wet mount may show WBCs.
Rx: Oral or intravaginal estrogen.

No
Consider: Allergic vaginitis. May be reaction to latex, detergents, spermacides, or vaginal hygiene products.
Rx: Avoid or remove offending agent

---

1. Metronidazole has antabuse effect – avoid ethanol; cannot use in 1st trimester pregnancy. Clindamycin: cannot use orally 1st trimester pregnancy
1998 Guidelines for Treatment of Sexually Transmitted Diseases. MMWR 1998; 47 (No RR-1).
Botash, AS., Howes, D. Vaginitis. June 24, 1998. Http://www.emedicine.enemg/topics631.htm.
Sobel, JD. Candidal Vulvovaginitis. Clinical Obst Gyn 1993; 38: 153-1685.
Fox, KK, Behets, FMT. Vaginal Discharge. Post Grad Med 1995; 95: 87-104.
Easmon, CSF, Hay, PE, Ison, CA. Bacterial Vaginosis: A Diagnostic Approach. Genitourin Med 1992; 68: 134-138.

83

8c: Urethral Discharge/Genital Ulcers

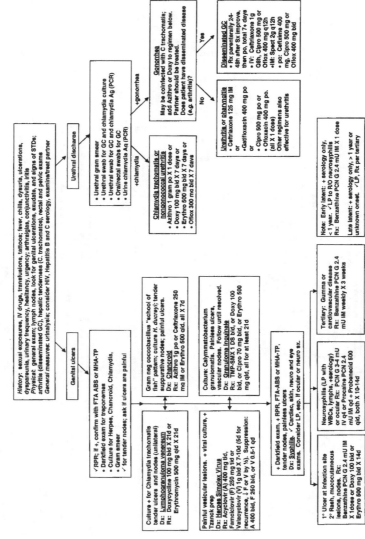

History: sexual exposures, IV drugs, transfusions, tattoos; fever, chills, dysuria, urinary frequency, hesitancy, urgency; arthralgias, conjunctivitis, iritis
Physical: general exam; lymph nodes, look for genital ulcerations, exudate, and signs of STDs; arthritis (disseminated GC); hepatic tenderness (C. trachomatis), rectal and pelvic exams
General measures: urinalysis; consider HIV, Hepatitis B and C serology, examine/treat partner

Genital ulcers

✓RPR; if +, confirm with FTA ABS or MHA-TP
• Darkfield exam for treponemes
• Culture for Herpes, Chancroid, Chlamydia,
• Gram smear
✓ for tender nodes; ask if ulcers are painful

Culture + for Chlamydia trachomatis tender ulcers and nodes (unilateral)
Dx: **Lymphogranuloma venereum**
Rx: Doxycycline 100 mg bid X 21d or Erythromycin 500 mg qid X 21d

Painful vesicular lesions. + viral culture, + Tzanck prep
Dx: **Herpes Simplex Virus**
Rx: Acyclovir (A) 400 mg bid,
Famciclovir (F) 250 mg tid or Valacyclovir (V) 1g qid X 7-10d (5d for recurrence), ↓ F or V by ½). Suppression: A 400 bid, F 250 bid, or V 0.5-1 qd

Gram neg coccobacillus "school of fish" pattern; culture *H. ducreyi*; tender suppurative nodes; painful ulcers.
Dx: **Chancroid**
Rx: Azithro 1g po or Ceftriaxone 250 mg IM or Erythro 500 qid, all X 7d

Culture: Calymmatobacterium granulomatis. Painless ulcers, vascular nodes. Follow until resolved.
Dx: **Granuloma Inguinale**
Rx: TMP-SMX 1 DS bid, or Doxy 100 bid, or Cipro 70 mg bid, or Erythro 500 mg qid, all for at least 21d

+ Darkfield exam, + RPR, FTA-ABS or MHA-TP, tender nodes, painless ulcers
Dx: **Syphilis**. ✓ Cardiac, skin, neuro and eye exams. Consider LP, esp. if ocular or neuro sx.

1° Ulcer at infection site
2° Rash, mucocutaneous lesions, nodes. Rx:
Benzathine PCN G 2.4 mU IM X 1 dose or Doxy 100 bid or Erythro 500 mg bid X 14d

Neurosyphilis (LP with WBCs, lymphs, +serology) or ocular Rx: PCN G 3-4 mU IV q4 or Procaine PCN 2.4 mU IM qd + Probenecid 500 qid, both X 10-14d

Tertiary: Gumma or cardiovascular disease Rx: Benzathine PCN G 2.4 mU IM weekly X 3 weeks

Note: Early latent: + serology only, < 1 year. ✓LP to R/O neurosyphilis
Rx: Benzathine PCN G 2.4 mU IM X 1 dose

Late latent: + serology only, > 1 year or unknown onset. ✓LP, Rx per tertiary

Urethral discharge

• Urethral gram smear
• Urethral swab for GC and chlamydia culture
• Urethral swab for GC and chlamydia Ag (PCR)
• Oral/rectal swabs for GC
• Urine chlamydia Ag (PCR)

+chlamydia

Chlamydia trachomatis or nongonococcal urethritis
• Azithro 1 gram po X 1 dose or
• Doxy 100 mg bid X 7 days or
• Erytho 500 mg bid X 7 days or
• Oflox 300 mg bid X 7 days

+gonorrhea

Gonorrhea
May be coinfected with C trachomatis; add Azithro or Doxy to regimen below. Partner should be treated. Does patient have disseminated disease (e.g. arthritis)?

No → **Urethritis or pharyngitis**
• Ceftriaxone 125 mg IM or
• Gatifloxacin 400 mg po or
• Cipro 500 mg po or
• Ofloxacin 400 mg po. (all X 1 dose)
Other regimens also effective for urethritis

Yes → **Disseminated GC**
• Rx parenterally 24-48h after Sx improve, then po, total 7+ days
• IV: Ceftriaxone 1g Q8h, Cipro 500 mg or Oflox 400 mg q12h
• IM: Spect 2g q12h
• po: Cefixime 400 mg, Cipro 500 mg or Oflox 400 mg bid

Azithro – azithromycin, PCN –penicillin; doxy– doxycycline, erythro –erythromycin, mU – million units, cipro – ciprofloxacin, oflox – ofloxacin, spect – spectinomycin
1998 Guidelines for Treatment of Sexually Transmitted Diseases. MMWR Vol 47 No. RR-1, January 23, 1998.
Keiger, JN, New Sexually Transmitted Disease Treatment Guidelines, Infections in Urology 1998; 154:209-213.
Simmons, P. Non-Specific Urethritis. The Practitioner. 1993;237; 624-628
Elrod, Walter. Urethritis, Male. URL: http://www.emedicine.com/EMERG/topic623.htm

8d: Hematuria

Generally defined as greater than 2 RBC's / HPF. Some suggest any RBCs are significant.
• R/O false positive: hypochlorite, menstrual blood, sexual trauma, medications (chloroquine, L-dopa, methyldopa, nitrofurantoin, phenolphthalein laxatives, phenazopyridine, phenothiazines, pyridium phenytoin, quinine, rifampin), myoglobin (hemolysis), hemoglobin (hemolysis), prophyria, high specific gravity, beets and rhubarb.
• Hx with attention to: trauma, upper respiratory infection (post-streptococcal GN), skin infection (post-streptococcal GN), hemoptysis (Goodpasture's, Wegener's), family history (familial hematuria, Alport's (deafness), sickle cell disease/trait, coagulopathy, urolithiasis, cystic renal disease), porphyria, exercise (benign exercise induced hematuria), medications (anticoagulants, analgesics, cyclophosphamide), renal stones, vasculitis, prior hepatitis B or C, smoker, toxins (bladder tumor), trauma, endometriosis, travel (schistosomiasis), pelvic irradiation.
• PE with attention to ecchymosis, blood pressure (reno-vascular), rash (IgA nephropathy, SLE, Henoch-Schönlein purpura), flank bruit (reno-vascular, A-V fistula), evidence of endocarditis, BPH

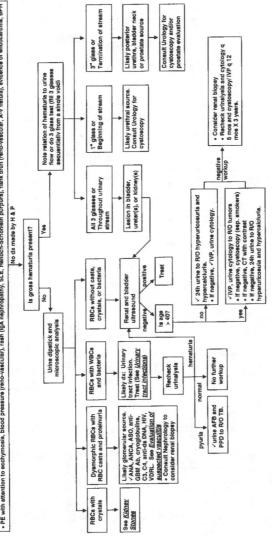

Schaeffer AJ, Del Greco F. Other renal diseases of urologic significance. In: Walsh, PC, Retik, AB, Stamey, TA, Vaughan, ED (ed), Campbell's Urology, pp 2065-72, W. B. Saunders 1992.
Kanarvogel, LE. Common urinary symptoms: Hematuria. In: Rakel, RE (editor), Sanders Manual of Medical Practice. pp 518-519. W. B. Saunders, 1996
Ahmed Z, Lee J. Asymptomatic urinary abnormalities: Hematuria and Proteinuria. Med Clin NA 1997: 81: 641-649
Sparwasser C, Cimmiak HU, Treiber U, Pust RA. Significance of the evaluation of asymptomatic microscopic haematuria in young men. BJ Urol 1994; 74: 723-729.
Rockall AG, Newman-Sanders APG, Al-Kutoubi MA, Vale JA. Haematuria. Postgrad Med J 1997; 73: 129-136
Fracchia JA, Motta J, Miller LS, et al. Evaluation of asymptomatic microhematuria. Urology 1996; 48:484-489.

8e: Lower Urinary Tract Symptoms and Benign Prostatic Hyperplasia (BPH)

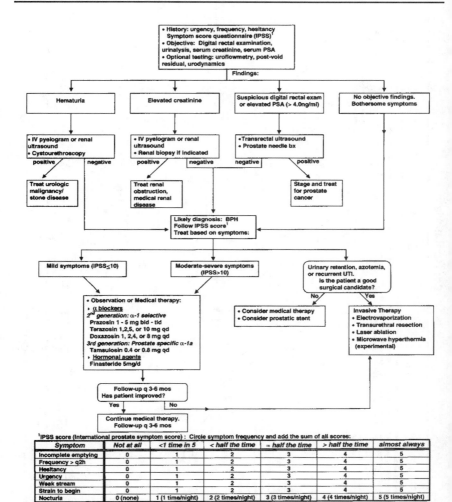

- History: urgency, frequency, hesitancy
  Symptom score questionnaire (IPSS)[1]
- Objective: Digital rectal examination,
  urinalysis, serum creatinine, serum PSA
- Optional testing: uroflowmetry, post-void
  residual, urodynamics

Findings:

Hematuria	Elevated creatinine	Suspicious digital rectal exam or elevated PSA (> 4.0ng/ml)	No objective findings. Bothersome symptoms

- IV pyelogram or renal ultrasound
- Cystourethroscopy

positive / negative

Treat urologic malignancy/ stone disease

- IV pyelogram or renal ultrasound
- Renal biopsy if indicated

positive / negative

Treat renal obstruction, medical renal disease

- Transrectal ultrasound
- Prostate needle bx

negative / positive

Stage and treat for prostate cancer

Likely diagnosis: BPH
Follow IPSS score[1]
Treat based on symptoms:

Mild symptoms (IPSS≤10)	Moderate-severe symptoms (IPSS>10)	Urinary retention, azotemia, or recurrent UTI. Is the patient a good surgical candidate?

- Observation or Medical therapy:
  - α blockers
    2nd generation: α-1 selective
    Prazosin 1 - 5 mg bid - tid
    Terazosin 1,2,5, or 10 mg qd
    Doxazosin 1, 2,4, or 8 mg qd
    3rd generation: Prostate specific α-1a
    Tamsulosin 0.4 or 0.8 mg qd
  - Hormonal agents
    Finasteride 5mg/d

No / Yes

- Consider medical therapy
- Consider prostatic stent

Invasive Therapy
- Electrovaporization
- Transurethral resection
- Laser ablation
- Microwave hyperthermia (experimental)

Follow-up q 3-6 mos
Has patient improved?

Yes / No

Continue medical therapy.
Follow-up q 3-6 mos

[1]IPSS score (International prostate symptom score) : Circle symptom frequency and add the sum of all scores:

Symptom	Not at all	<1 time in 5	< half the time	= half the time	> half the time	almost always
Incomplete emptying	0	1	2	3	4	5
Frequency > q2h	0	1	2	3	4	5
Hesitancy	0	1	2	3	4	5
Urgency	0	1	2	3	4	5
Weak stream	0	1	2	3	4	5
Strain to begin	0	1	2	3	4	5
Nocturia	0 (none)	1 (1 time/night)	2 (2 times/night)	3 (3 times/night)	4 (4 times/night)	5 (5 times/night)

Barry MJ, Fowler FJ, O'Leary MP et al. and Measurement Committee of the American Urological Association: The American Urological Association symptom index for benign prostatic hyperplasia. J. Urol 148: 1549, 1992

9a: Anemia

The etiology of most anemias in adults is easily definable with a careful history, physical, and a minimum of diagnostic studies. However, these studies must be obtained prior to transfusion or initiation of therapy. There are in essence, only two causes of anemia: failure of production and increased destruction. Two readily obtainable pieces of information are all that are required to determine further work-up: (1) Classification of anemia: MCV and (2) Evaluation of marrow response: reticulocyte index (RI). RI = % reticulocytes X patient Hct/normal Hct. Divide RI by 2 if polychromasia is present.

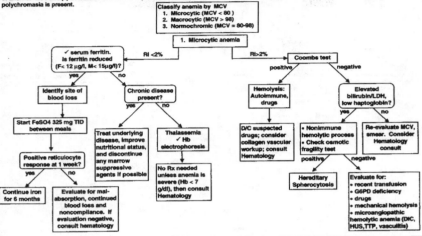

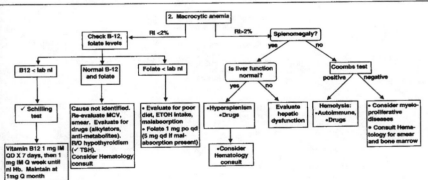

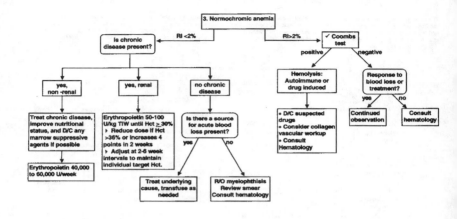

Summary

The common causes of microcytic anemia:
- Iron deficiency
- Thalassemia
- Chronic disease

The common causes of macrocytic anemia:
- B-12 and folate deficiency
- Liver disease
- Reticulocytosis

The common causes of normochromic anemia:
- Chronic disease
- Early acute blood loss
- Intrinsic defects

9b: Workup of the Patient with Bleeding Disorder

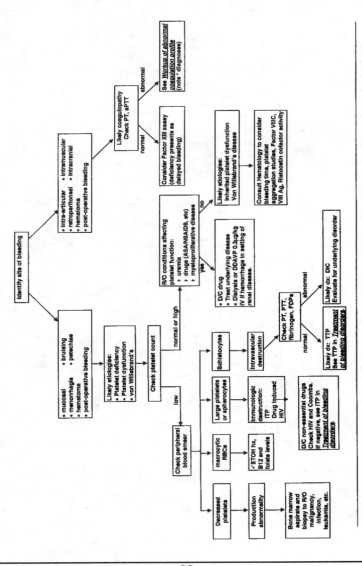

Coller BS and Schneiderman Pl. Clinical evaluation of hemorrhagic disorders: Bleeding history and differential diagnosis of purpura. In Hoffman R, Benz EJ, Shattil SJ, Furie B, Cohen HJ, and Silberstein LE eds., Hematology, Basic Principles and Practice, Churchill Livingstone, New York 1995 p. 1906-1622.

9c: Workup of the Patient with Hypercoagulable State

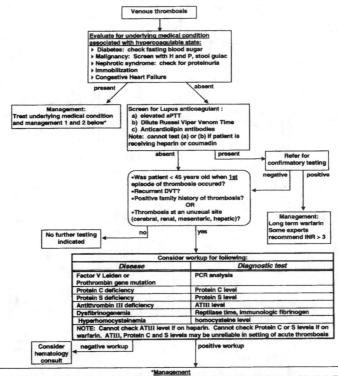

```
                    ┌─────────────────────┐
                    │  Venous thrombosis  │
                    └─────────────────────┘
```

Evaluate for underlying medical condition associated with hypercoagulable state:
- Diabetes: check fasting blood sugar
- Malignancy: Screen with H and P, stool guiac
- Nephrotic syndrome: check for proteinuria
- Immobilization
- Congestive Heart Failure

present → / absent →

Management:
Treat underlying medical condition and management 1 and 2 below*

Screen for Lupus anticoagulant :
a) elevated aPTT
b) Dilute Russel Viper Venom Time
c) Anticardiolipin antibodies
Note: cannot test (a) or (b) if patient is receiving heparin or coumadin

absent / present → **Refer for confirmatory testing** (negative / positive)

- Was patient < 45 years old when 1st episode of thrombosis occured?
- Recurrent DVT?
- Positive family history of thrombosis?
  OR
- Thrombosis at an unusual site (cerebral, renal, mesenteric, hepatic)?

Management:
Long term warfarin
Some experts recommend INR > 3

no → **No further testing indicated** / yes

Consider workup for following:

Disease	Diagnostic test
Factor V Leiden or Prothrombin gene mutation	PCR analysis
Protein C deficiency	Protein C level
Protein S deficiency	Protein S level
Antithrombin III deficiency	ATIII level
Dysfibrinogenemia	Reptilase time, immunologic fibrinogen
Hyperhomocysteinemia	homocysteine level

NOTE: Cannot check ATIII level if on heparin. Cannot check Protein C or S levels if on warfarin. ATIII, Protein C and S levels may be unreliable in setting of acute thrombosis

negative workup → **Consider hematology consult** / positive workup

***Management**
1. Long term warfarin therapy is recommended if a patient has: (a) more than one thrombotic event or (b) a single life threatening event
2. Prophylactic or treatment anticoagulation regimens (see *Prophylaxis for Deep Venous Thrombosis*) are suggested if a patient will undergo a procedure that may be thrombogenic
3. Consider DVT prophylaxis with heparin if pregnant

Note: Pregnant women with thrombosis should be treated with heparin. They should not receive warfarin.

1. Schulman S, Grandqvist S, Holmstrom M, et al. The duration of oral anticoagulation therapy after a second episode of venous thromboembolism. N Engl J Med 336: 393-8, 1997
2. DeStefano V, Finazzi G, Mannucci PM. Inherited Thrombophilia: pathogenesis, clinical syndromes, and management. Blood 87: 3531-3544, 1996
3. Bauer KA. Management of patients with hereditary defects predisposing to thrombosis including pregnant women. Thrombosis and Haemostasis 74:94-100, 1995

9d: Workup of Abnormal Coagulation Profile

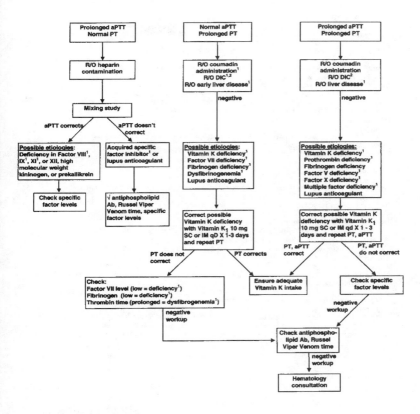

1. Associated with bleeding disorders
2. ✓ platelet count, fibrinogen, fibrin degradation products

Santoro SA and Eby CS. Laboratory evaluation of hemostatic disorders. In Hoffman R, Benz EJ, Shattil SJ, Furie B, Cohen HJ, and Silberstein LE eds., Hematology, Basic Principles and Practice, Churchill Livingstone, New York 1995 p. 1622-1632

Thrombocytopenia: Production abnormality (hematology consult recommended)
• Patient not actively bleeding: Transfuse platelets only if less than 10,000 (some recommend 20,000)
• Patient actively bleeding: Transfuse if platelet count is less than 50,000

Thrombocytopenia: Destruction abnormality (hematology consult recommended)
• TTP: Plasmapheresis
• ITP: Steroids: - prednisone 1mg/kg/day; taper when plt > 100,000
            - IV Gamma Globulin: 0.4 g/kg/day X 5 days or 1 g/kg/day X 2 days
            - Splenectomy: if unresponsive to glucocorticoids (give pneumococcal, meningococcal, and H influenza vaccinations prior to splenectomy)

Vitamin K deficiency:
• Vitamin K_1 10 mg QD X 1-3 days IM or SC. Patients at risk (e.g. on TPN), should receive prophylactic treatment with vitamin K_1 10 mg po or SC TIW.
• Fresh Frozen Plasma: 2-4 units IV if patient is bleeding

Warfarin overdose
• Hold warfarin
• Low dose Vitamin K_1, 1 mg po or SC, if patient needs to remain therapeutic on warfarin
• Vitamin K_1 10 mg IM or SC if hemorrhage present or full correction desired
• Fresh Frozen Plasma: 2-4 units IV if hemorrhage present

von Willebrand's Disease
• Desmopressin acetate: 0.3 µg/kg IV. May be repeated Q 24H; tachyphylaxis may occur
• Virally inactivated von Willebrand Factor concentrate
• Cryoprecipitate: 10 bags (if life or limb threatening emergency and virally inactivated concentrate is not available)
• Consult Hematology

Factor deficiencies

Multiple factor deficiency:	fresh frozen plasma
Fibrinogen deficiency:	Cryoprecipitate
Factor VIII deficiency:	virus inactivated Factor VIII concentrate, 50u/kg load for 100% replacement
Factor IX deficiency	virus inactivated Factor IX concentrate, 80-100 u/kg load for 100% replacement
Factor XI deficiency:	fresh frozen plasma (Factor XI concentrate NA in USA)

9f: Management of Emergent Transfusion Reactions

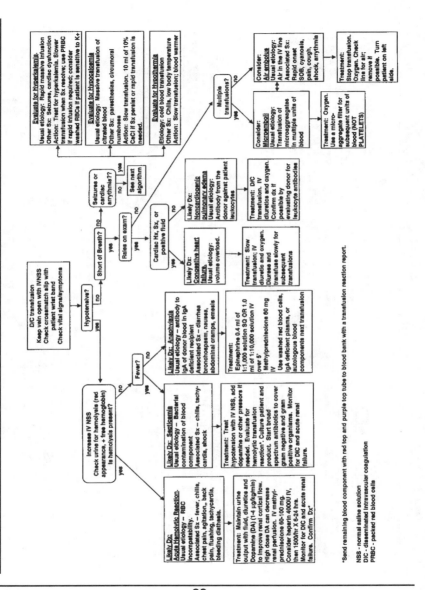

D/C transfusion
Keep vein open with IV NSS
Check crossmatch slip with patient wrist band
Check vital signs/symptoms

Increase IV NSS
Check urine for hemolysis (red appearance, + free hemoglobin)
Is hemolysis present?

yes

Likely Dx: Acute Hemolytic Reaction.
Usual etiology – RBC incompatibility.
Associated Sx – fever, chills, chest pain, agitation, back pain, flushing, tachycardia, bleeding diathesis.

Treatment: Maintain urine output with fluid, diuretics and Dopamine (DA) (1-4 µg/kg/min) to improve renal cortical flow. High dose DA can decrease renal perfusion. IV methyl-prednisolone 60-100 mg IV. Consider heparin 4000U IV, then 1500/hr X 6-24 hrs. Monitor for DIC and acute renal failure. Confirm Dx*

Fever?

yes

Likely Dx: Septicemia
Usual etiology – Bacterial contamination of blood component.
Associated Sx – chills, tachycardia, shock

Treatment: Treat hypotension with IV NSS, add dopamine or other pressors if needed. Evaluate for hemolytic transfusion reaction*. Culture patient and product. Start broad spectrum antibiotics to cover gram negative and gram positive organisms. Monitor for DIC and acute renal failure.

no

Hypotensive?

yes → **Fever?** (see above) / **no**

Likely Dx: Anaphylaxis
Usual etiology – antibody to IgA of donor blood in IgA deficient recipient
Associated Sx – diarrhea, bronchospasm, nausea, abdominal cramps, emesis

Treatment:
Epinephrine 0.4 ml of 1:1,000 solution SQ OR 1.0 ml of 1:10,000 solution IV over 5'
Methylprednisolone 60 mg IV
Use washed red blood cells, IgA deficient plasma, or autologous blood components next transfusion

no

Short of Breath?

yes → **Rales on exam?**

yes → **Cardiac Hx, Sx, or positive fluid**

yes

Likely Dx: Congestive heart failure.
Usual etiology: volume overload.

Treatment: Slow transfusion; IV diuretic and oxygen. Diuresis and transfuse slowly for subsequent transfusions

no

Likely Dx: Noncardiogenic pulmonary edema
Usual etiology: Antibody from the donor against patient leukocytes

Treatment: D/C transfusion, IV diuretics and oxygen. Confirm dx if possible by evaluating donor for leukocyte antibodies

no (Rales on exam? → no)

Seizures or cardiac arrythmia??

yes

Evaluate for Hyperkalemia.
Usual etiology: Rapid massive infusion
Other Sx: Seizures, cardiac dysfunction
Action: Treat for hyperkalemia. Slower transfusion when Sx resolve; use PRBC if rapid infusion required; consider washed RBCs if patient is sensitive to K+

Evaluate for Hypocalcemia
Usual etiology: Massive transfusion of citrated blood
Other Sx: paresthesias, circumoral numbness
Action: Slow transfusion. 10 ml of 10% CaCl if Sx persist or rapid transfusion is needed.

no → See next algorithm

no (Short of Breath? → no)

Multiple transfusions?

yes

Evaluate for Hypothermia
Etiology: cold blood transfusion
Other Sx: Chills, low body temperature
Action: Slow transfusion; blood warmer

Consider:
Air embolus
Usual etiology: Air in the IV line
Associated Sx: Rapid onset SOB, cyanosis, shock, arrythmia

Treatment: Stop transfusion. Oxygen. Check line for air; remove if possible. Turn patient on left side.

Consider:
Microemboli
Usual etiology: Transfusion of microaggregates in multiple units of blood

Treatment: Oxygen. Use a micro-aggregate filter for subsequent units of blood (NOT PLATELETS)

*Send remaining blood component with red top and purple top tube to blood bank with a transfusion reaction report.

NSS – normal saline solution
DIC – disseminated intravascular coagulation
PRBC – packed red blood cells

93

9g: Management of Nonemergent Transfusion Reactions

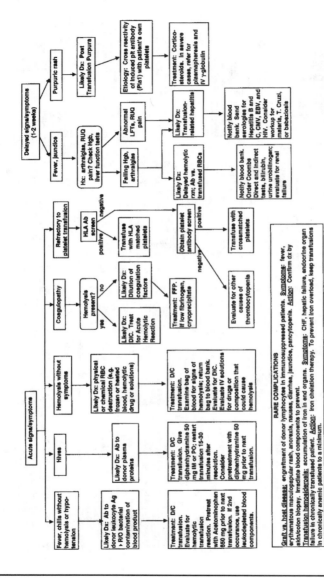

Acute signs/symptoms

Fever, chills without hemolysis or hypotension
Likely Dx: Ab to donor leukocyte Ag > R/O bacterial contamination of blood product
Treatment: D/C transfusion. Evaluate for hemolytic reaction. Pretreat with Acetominophen 650 mg prior to next transfusion. If 2nd occurrence, use leukodepleted blood components.

Hives
Likely Dx: Ab to donor plasma proteins
Treatment: D/C transfusion. Give diphenhydramine 50 mg IM or PO; restart transfusion 15-30 minutes after resolution. Consider pretreatment with diphenhydramine 50 mg prior to next transfusion.

Hemolysis without symptoms
Likely Dx: physical or chemical RBC destruction (e.g. frozen or heated blood, hemolytic drug or solutions)
Treatment: D/C transfusion. Examine bag of blood for signs of hemolysis; return bag to blood bank. Evaluate for DIC. Evaluate IV solutions for drugs or composition that could cause hemolysis.

Coagulopathy
Hemolysis present?
- yes → Likely Dx: DIC. Treat for Acute Hemolytic Reaction
- no → Likely Dx: Dilution of coagulation factors → Treatment: FFP. If low fibrinogen, cryoprecipitate

Refractory to platelet transfusion
HLA Ab screen
- positive → Transfuse with HLA matched platelets
- negative → Obtain platelet antibody screen
  - positive → Transfuse with crossmatched platelets
  - negative → Evaluate for other causes of thrombocytopenia

Delayed signs/symptoms (1-2 weeks)

Purpuric rash
Likely Dx: Post Transfusion Purpura
Etiology: Cross reactivity of induced plt antibody (Plat) with patient's own platelets
Treatment: Corticosteroids. In severe cases, refer for plasmapheresis and IV γ-globulin

Fever, jaundice
Hx: arthralgias, RUQ pain? Check Hgb, liver function tests
- Abnormal LFTs, RUQ pain → Likely Dx: Transfusion-related hepatitis → Notify blood bank. Send serologies for Hepatitis B and C, CMV, EBV, and HIV. Consider workup for malaria, T. Cruzi, or babesiosis
- Falling Hgb, arthralgias → Likely Dx: Delayed hemolytic rxn; Ab via transfused RBCs → Notify blood bank. Order Coombs Direct and Indirect tests, bilirubin, urine urobilinogen; evaluate for renal failure

---

RARE COMPLICATIONS

Graft vs. host disease: engraftment of donor lymphocytes in immunosuppressed patients. **Symptoms:** fever, erythematous maculopapular rash, anorexia, nausea, diarrhea, jaundice, pancytopenia. **Action:** Confirm dx by skin/colon biopsy. Irradiate blood components to prevent.

Transfusion hemosiderosis: accumulation of iron in end organs. **Symptoms:** CHF, hepatic failure, endocrine organ failure in chronically transfused patient. **Action:** Iron chelation therapy. To prevent iron overload, keep transfusions to a minimum in chronically anemic patients.

Jenner PW and Holland PV. The diagnosis and management of transfusion reactions. In Clinical Practice of Transfusion Medicine, 3rd edition. Petz LD, Swisher SN, Kleinman S, Spence RK and Strauss RG eds. Churchill Livingstone, Chapter 41, 905-930, 1995

Circular of Information for the use of human blood and blood components. Am. Assoc. of Community Blood Centers,1995

Brecher ME, Greenberger PA, Stack G, Judge JV, Snyder EL, Roberts GT, and Secher RA. Transfusion reactions. In Principles of Transfusion Medicine, 2nd ed. Rossi EC, Simon TL, Moss GS, and Gould SA eds. Williams and Wilkins, Section XIV: Chapters 72-75, pp 747-802 1996

10a: Antiretroviral Therapy in HIV Disease[1]

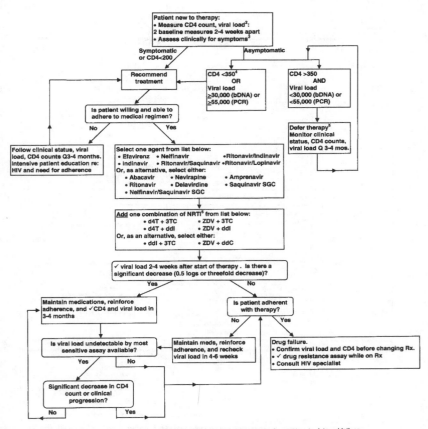

1. Recommendations change frequently. Check www.hivatis.org and www.pocketdoctor.com for most up to date guidelines.
2. Viral load should not be measured for four weeks after intercurrent infection/illness or immunization.
3. Thrush, unexplained fever, and those who have progressed from HIV+ status to AIDS.
4. Controversial. Clear <u>clinical</u> benefit of treatment demonstrated only for CD4 <200.
5. Controversial. Some experts advocate treatment in this situation.
6. NRTI= Nucleoside Reverse Transcriptase Inhibitor; ZDV = zidovudine; ddI = didanosine; ddC = zalcitabine; d4T = stavudine; 3TC = lamivudine. See table 1, <u>*Antiretroviral agents*</u> for dosages.

Department of Health and Human Services. Guidelines for the use of antiretroviral agents in HIV-infected adults and adolescents. HIV/AIDS Treatment Information Service, February 2001, www.hivatis.org. Also see www.pocketdoctor.com for updates.

10b: Antiretroviral Agents

Protease Inhibitors[1]

Drug	Dose (oral)	Considerations	Common side effects
Indinavir (Crixivan)	800 mg q 8hr	taken 1 hr before or 2 hrs after a meal Increase po fluids	nausea, abdominal pain, headache diarrhea, vomiting, nephrolithiasis, increased indirect bilirubin
Nelfinavir (Viracept)	750 mg tid or 1250 mg bid	taken with food	diarrhea, flatulence, nausea, rash
Ritonavir (Norvir)	600 mg q12h	taken with food Start with 200 mg q12h and gradually increase over 5-7 days to 600 q12h	nausea, diarrhea, vomiting, taste perversion, abdominal pain, circumoral paresthesia, increased triglycerides
Saquinavir HGC (Invirase)	400 mg po bid with Ritonavir (see below)	taken with a meal	diarrhea, nausea, abdominal pain, headache
Saquinavir SGC (Fortovase)	1200 mg tid	taken with a meal or up to 2hrs after	diarrhea, nausea, abdominal pain, dyspepsia, headache
Ritonavir + Saquinavir Combination	400 mg bid (R) 400 mg bid (S)	Dose same - HGC or SGC	As noted above
Amprenavir (Agenerase)	1200 mg bid		rash, diarrhea, nausea, vomiting, oral paresthesias
Lopinavir/ritonavir	400 mg(L)/100 mg (R) bid	take with food, ↑dose to 533/133 if used with efavirenz	diarrhea, nausea, abnormal stools, asthenia, hyperlipidemia
Ritonavir+Indinavir combination	200 mg (R)/800 mg (I) q12h or 400 mg (R)/400 mg (I) q12h	Can be taken with or without food. Increase po fluids	Increased incidence nephrolithiasis; see Indinavir and Ritonavir above

Nucleoside Reverse Transcriptase Inhibitors (NRTI)[2]

Drug	Dose (oral)	Considerations	Common side effects
Zidovudine (Retrovir, ZDV)	300 mg bid or 200 mg tid		anemia, neutropenia, GI intolerance, headache, insomnia, asthenia
Didanosine, (Videx, Videx EC, ddI)	>60 kg: 200mg bid or 400 mg qd, <60 kg: 125mg bid or 250 mg qd	take on empty stomach	pancreatitis, peripheral neuropathy, nausea, diarrhea
Zalcitabine, (HIVID, ddC)	0.75 mg tid		peripheral neuropathy, stomatitis
Stavudine (Zerit, d4T)	>60 kg: 40mg bid, <60kg: 30mg bid		peripheral neuropathy
Lamivudine, (Epivir, 3TC)	> 50 kg: 150 mg bid <50 kg: 2mg/kg bid		adverse effects uncommon, rarely headache, GI intolerance
Abacavir (Ziagen)[3]	300 mg bid	3% of patients develop hypersensitivity reaction[3]	Headache, nausea

Non-Nucleoside Reverse Transcriptase Inhibitors (NNRTI)

Drug	Dose (oral)	Considerations	Common side effects
Nevirapine (Viramune)	200 mg bid	Start with 200 mg qd for first 14 days	rash, increased transaminases, hepatitis
Delavirdine(Rescriptor)	400 mg tid		rash, headaches
Efavirenz (Sustiva)	600 mg qd	Usually dosed qhs due to initial side effects. False positive cannabinoid test	Initial dizziness, lightheadedness, insomnia, rash

1. All protease inhibitors may cause worsening glycemic control in patients with diabetes mellitus or new onset diabetes mellitus. They may also cause fat redistribution and lipid abnormalities.
2. Lactic acidosis with hepatic steatosis may occur (rarely) with any NRTI and be life threatening.
3. Abacavir should be stopped as soon as a hypersensitivity reaction is suspected. Symptoms include fever, malaise, nausea, cough, vomiting, abdominal pain, or occasional rash. Resolves within 2 days of stopping medication. DO NOT restart as symptoms may worsen and lead to death. Read package insert. Report reaction to Abacavir Hypersensitivity Registry at: 1-800-270-0425.

Department of Health and Human Services. Guidelines for the use of antiretroviral agents in HIV-infected adults and adolescents. HIV/AIDS Treatment Information Service, February 2001, www.hivatis.org.

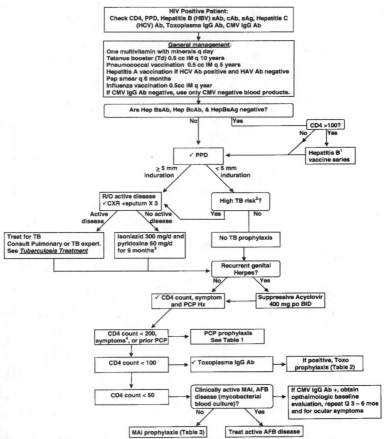

HIV Positive Patient:
Check CD4, PPD, Hepatitis B (HBV) sAb, cAb, sAg, Hepatitis C (HCV) Ab, Toxoplasma IgG Ab, CMV IgG Ab

General management:
One multivitamin with minerals q day
Tetanus booster (Td) 0.5 cc IM q 10 years
Pneumococcal vaccination 0.5 cc IM q 5 years
Hepatitis A vaccination if HCV Ab positive and HAV Ab negative
Pap smear q 6 months
Influenza vaccination 0.5cc IM q year
If CMV IgG Ab negative, use only CMV negative blood products.

Are Hep BsAb, Hep BcAb, & HepBsAg negative?

No / Yes

CD4 >100?
No / Yes

Hepatitis B[1] vaccine series

✓ PPD

≥ 5 mm induration / < 5 mm induration

R/O active disease
✓CXR +sputum X 3

High TB risk[2]?
Yes / No

Active disease / No active disease

Treat for TB
Consult Pulmonary or TB expert.
See *Tuberculosis Treatment*

Isoniazid 300 mg/d and pyridoxine 50 mg/d for 9 months[3]

No TB prophylaxis

Recurrent genital Herpes?
No / Yes

Suppressive Acyclovir 400 mg po BID

✓ CD4 count, symptom and PCP Hx

CD4 count < 200, symptoms[4], or prior PCP

PCP prophylaxis
See Table 1

CD4 count < 100

✓ Toxoplasma IgG Ab

If positive, Toxo prophylaxis (Table 2)

CD4 count < 50

Clinically active MAI, AFB disease (mycobacterial blood culture)?
No / Yes

If CMV IgG Ab +, obtain opthalmologic baseline evaluation, repeat Q 3 – 6 mos and for ocular symptoms

MAI prophylaxis (Table 3)

Treat active AFB disease

1. Hepatitis B vaccine series : 3 IM doses, 20 mcg/dose at 0, 1 and 6 months. Benefit doubted with CD4 < 100 due to poor antibody response.
2. High risk: exposure to TB, injection drug user, homeless persons, and migrant workers.
3. Requires monthly clinical monitoring and liver transaminases at 1 and 3 months; alternative short course regimens are available.
4. Recurrent mucosal candidiasis, unexplained fevers ≥ 2 weeks, history AIDS defining illness

Centers for Disease Control and Prevention. 1999 USPHS/IDSA guidelines for the prevention of opportunistic infections in persons infected with human immunodeficiency virus. MMWR 48 (No. RR-10), 1999
Centers for Disease Control and Prevention. Prevention and treatment of tuberculosis among patients infected with human immunodeficiency virus: principles of therapy and revised recommendations. MMWR 47 (No. RR-20), 1998

10d: HIV Post-Exposure Prophylaxis (PEP)[1]

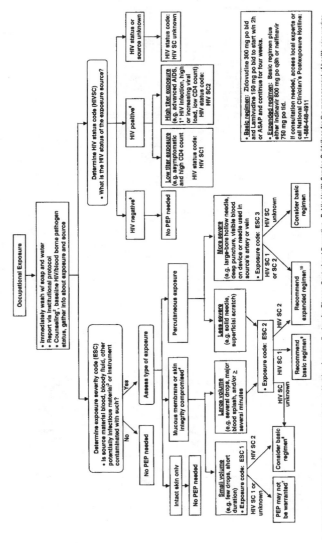

1. Adapted from and should be used in consultation with this reference: Centers for Disease Control and Prevention. Public Health Service Guidelines for the management of health care worker exposures to HIV and recommendations for post-exposure prophylaxis. MMWR 47 (No RR-7), 1998
2. Counseling to include: exposure risk, post exposure prophylaxis, safer sex methods, recommended precautions including avoidance of blood/organ donation, pregnancy and breast feeding.
3. Other potentially infectious material includes semen, vaginal secretions, cerebrospinal, synovial, pleural, peritoneal, pericardial or amniotic fluids; or tissue
4. Skin integrity compromised if chapped skin, dermatitis, abrasion, or open wound
5. Source considered HIV negative if negative HIV Ab, HIV by PCR, or HIV p24 Ag test performed at or near time of exposure and no evidence of recent retroviral-like illness.
6. Source considered HIV positive if positive lab test for HIV Ab, HIV by PCR, or HIV p24 Ag, or physician-diagnosed AIDS.
7. Exposure doesn't pose known risk for HIV transmission. Whether risk of drug toxicity outweighs benefit of PEP decided by exposed health care worker (HCW) and clinician.
8. Negligible risk of transmission based on exposure. High HIV titer in source may justify PEP. Whether risk of drug toxicity outweighs benefit of PEP decided by exposed HCW and clinician.
9. No risk of HIV transmission has been observed but PEP is appropriate.
10. Exposure indicates increased HIV transmission risk.

10e: Prophylactic Drugs for Adults with HIV Infection

All listed in order of preference
All are given orally unless otherwise specified

Table 1: PCP prophylaxis[1]

Drug	Dose	Side effects	Comments
TMP/SMX	1DS qd, or 1SS qd, or 1DS tiw	Nausea, vomiting, pruritis, rash, cytopenias, fever, elevated transaminases	• Clearly drug of choice • Many advocate desensitization for allergy • Provides concomitant bacterial and toxoplasmosis (toxo) prophylaxis.
Dapsone	100 mg qd	Rash, pruritis, hepatitis, anemia, neutropenia, Hemolytic anemia w/wo G6PD deficiency	• Provides concomitant toxo prophylaxis w/pyrimethamine 50 mg/wk & folinic acid 25 mg/wk. • ✓ for G6PD deficiency before use.
Pentamidine, aerosolized	300 mg q month via Respigard II nebulizer	Cough, wheeze, laryngitis, chest pain, dyspnea	Associated with atypical PCP presentation and greater failure rate
Atovaquone	750 mg bid	Diarrhea, rash	• Take with food • Provides concomitant toxo prophylaxis

Table 2: Toxoplasma prophylaxis - goal is to use one single regimen for PCP and toxo

Regimens	Dose	Side effects	Comments
TMP/SMX	1 DS qd, or 1 SS qd	See Table 1 above	• Regimen of choice. • Provides concomitant PCP prophylaxis.
Dapsone Pyrimethamine Folinic acid	50 mg qd 50 mg q wk 25 mg q wk	Marrow suppression, GI intolerance	• Provides concomitant PCP prophylaxis

Table 3: MAI prophylaxis[2]

Drug	Dose	Side effects	Comments
Azithromycin	1200 mg (single dose) q wk	GI intolerance, diarrhea	• Most cost-effective regimen. Concommittant bacterial prophylaxis
Clarithromycin	500 mg bid	GI intolerance, headache, transaminase elevation	Concommittant bacterial prophylaxis
Rifabutin	300 mg qd	Orange urine, rash, GI intolerance, neutropenia, dose related uveitis	Generally not used because of drug interactions. Dosage must be adjusted with many drugs including protease inhibitors and NNRTIs.

1. May discontinue primary prophylaxis if patient has sustained CD4 count > 200 for at least 3-6 months on antiretroviral therapy with sustained suppression of viral load

2. May consider discontinuing prophylaxis in patients with sustained CD4 count > 100 for 3-6 months and sustained suppression of viral load.

Abbreviations: PCP = pneumocystis carinii pneumonia; TMP/SMX = trimethoprim-sulfamethoxazole; DS = double strength; SS = single strength; toxo = toxoplasmosis; G6PD = glucose-6-phosphate dehydrogenase; tiw = three times/week; q wk = once a week

Centers for Disease Control and Prevention. 1999 USPHS/IDSA guidelines for the prevention of opportunistic infections in persons infected with human immunodeficiency virus. MMWR. 48(No. RR-10), 1999

11a: Initial Diagnostic Approach to Acute Low Back Pain

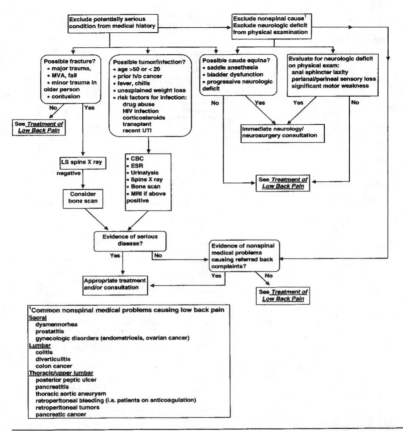

```
┌─────────────────────────┐          ┌──────────────────────────────┐
│ Exclude potentially      │          │ Exclude nonspinal cause¹      │
│ serious condition from   │─────────▶│ Exclude neurologic deficit    │
│ medical history          │          │ from physical examination     │
└─────────────────────────┘          └──────────────────────────────┘
```

Possible fracture?
- major trauma,
- MVA, fall
- minor trauma in older person
- contusion

No / Yes

See Treatment of Low Back Pain

Possible tumor/infection?
- age >50 or < 20
- prior h/o cancer
- fever, chills
- unexplained weight loss
- risk factors for infection:
  drug abuse
  HIV infection
  corticosteroids
  transplant
  recent UTI

Possible cauda equina?
- saddle anesthesia
- bladder dysfunction
- progressive neurologic deficit

No   Yes

Evaluate for neurologic deficit on physical exam:
anal sphincter laxity
perianal/perineal sensory loss
significant motor weakness

Yes   No

Immediate neurology/neurosurgery consultation

LS spine X ray

negative

Consider bone scan

- CBC
- ESR
- Urinalysis
- Spine X ray
- Bone scan
- MRI if above positive

See Treatment of Low Back Pain

Evidence of serious disease?

Yes   No

Evidence of nonspinal medical problems causing referred back complaints?

Yes   No

Appropriate treatment and/or consultation

See Treatment of Low Back Pain

---

¹Common nonspinal medical problems causing low back pain

Sacral
  dysmennorhea
  prostatitis
  gynecologic disorders (endometriosis, ovarian cancer)

Lumbar
  colitis
  diverticulitis
  colon cancer

Thoracic/upper lumbar
  posterior peptic ulcer
  pancreatitis
  thoracic aortic aneurysm
  retroperitoneal bleeding (i.e. patients on anticoagulation)
  retroperitoneal tumors
  pancreatic cancer

Bigos S, Bowyer O, Braen G, et al. Acute Low Back Problems in Adults. Clinical Practice Guideline, Quick Reference Guide Number. 14. Rockville, MD: U.S. Department of Health and Human Services, Public Health Service, Agency for Health Care Policy and Research, AHCPR Pub. No. 95-0643, December 1994.

11b: Treatment of Low Back Pain

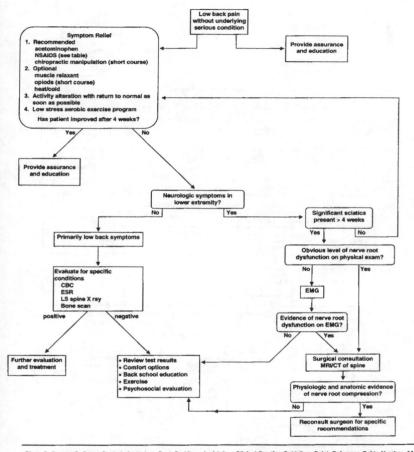

Bigos S, Bowyer O, Braen G, et al. Acute Low Back Problems in Adults. Clinical Practice Guideline, Quick Reference Guide Number. 14. Rockville, MD: U.S. Department of Health and Human Services, Public Health Service, Agency for Health Care Policy and Research, AHCPR Pub. No. 95-0643, December 1994.

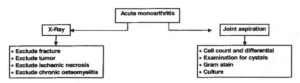

Acute monoarthritis

X-Ray

- Exclude fracture
- Exclude tumor
- Exclude ischemic necrosis
- Exclude chronic osteomyelitis

Joint aspiration

- Cell count and differential
- Examination for cystals
- Gram stain
- Culture

Types of Joint Effusions

Criteria	Normal	Non-inflammatory	Inflammatory	Purulent	Hemorrhagic
1. volume	<3.5 ml	often >3.5 ml	often>3.5 ml	>3.5 ml	>3.5 ml
2. color	clear	xanthochromic	xanthochromic to white	depends on organism	bloody
3. clarity	transparent	transparent	translucent to opaque	opaque	bloody
4. viscosity	high	high	low	variable	like blood
5. mucin clot	firm	firm	friable	friable	
6. clot	no	occasional	often	often	
7. WBC(mm3)	<200	200-2000	2000-100,000 (20,000 average)	>50,000	blood
8. % polys	<25%	<25%	>75%	>75%	blood
9. culture	Neg	Neg	Neg	Pos or Neg	Neg

Differential Diagnosis of Joint Effusions

Non-inflammatory	Inflammatory	Purulent	Hemorrhagic
Osteoarthritis	Rheumatoid arthritis	Bacterial infection	Trauma
Trauma	Reiter's syndrome	Acute gout	Fracture
Osteochondritis	Acute crystal synovitis		Blood dyscrasia
Avascular necrosis	Psoriatic arthritis		Charcot joint
SLE	Enteropathic arthritis		Pigmented villonodular synovitis
Amyloidosis	Lyme Disease		Tumor
Chronic crystal synovitis	Viral arthritis		
	Rheumatic fever		
	Infectious arthritis		
	bacterial		
	tuberculosis		
	fungal		

Aspiration of Inflammatory or Purulent Fluid from Monoarthritis

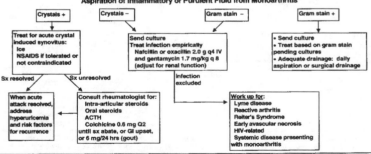

Crystals +

Treat for acute crystal induced synovitus:
  Ice
  NSAIDS if tolerated or not contraindicated

Sx resolved   Sx unresolved

When acute attack resolved, address hyperuricemia and risk factors for recurrence

Consult rheumatologist for:
  Intra-articular steroids
  Oral steroids
  ACTH
  Colchicine 0.6 mg Q2 until sx abate, or GI upset, or 6 mg/24 hrs (gout)

Crystals −

Send culture
Treat infection empirically
Nafcillin or oxacillin 2.0 g q4 IV and gentamycin 1.7 mg/kg q 8 (adjust for renal function)

Gram stain −

infection excluded

Work up for:
Lyme disease
Reactive arthritis
Reiter's Syndrome
Early avascular necrosis
HIV-related
Systemic disease presenting with monoarthritis

Gram stain +

- Send culture
- Treat based on gram stain pending cultures
- Adequate drainage: daily aspiration or surgical drainage

1. Baker, DG and Schumacher, HR. Acute Monoarthritis. NEJM 329:1013-1020, 1993.
2. Emmerson, BT. The Management of Gout. NEJM. 334:445-451, 1996.

11d: Table of Nonsteroidal Anti-Inflammatory Drugs (NSAIDs)

Salicylates

Generic	Brand name	Dose Range (mg/day)*	Dose Interval	Comments
Acetylsalicylic acid	Aspirin	1000-6000	q.i.d.	

Nonacetylated salicylates

Generic	Brand name	Dose Range (mg/day)*	Dose Interval	Comments
Choline magnesium trisalicylate	Trilisate	1500-3000	b.i.d. to t.i.d.	Liquid available Salicylate levels available
Salicylsalicylic acid	Disalcid	1500-3000	b.i.d. to t.i.d.	Salicylate levels available
	Salflex	1500-3000	b.i.d. to t.i.d.	Salicylate levels available

Nonacetylated salicylates have decreased effects on platelets, gastric mucosa and prostaglandin mediated renal function as compared to acetylsalicylic acid. They are generally considered safe in aspirin-sensitive asthma.

Short Serum Half Life NSAIDs

Generic	Brand name	Dose Range (mg/day)*	Dose Interval	Comments
Diclofenac potassium	Cataflam	100-200	bid to tid	Monitor ALT (SGPT) within
Diclofenac sodium	Voltaran	100-200	bid to tid	4 – 8 weeks
Diclofenac sodium with misoprostel	Arthrotec	200 – 300	Bid	200 mcg misoprostol coating
Fenoprofen calcium	Nalfon	1200-3200	tid to qid	Acute interstitial nephritis
Flurbiprofen	Ansaid	100-300	bid to qid	
Ibuprofen	Motrin	1200-3200	tid to qid	Liquid available
Ketoprofen	Orudis	150-300	tid to qid	
	Oruvail	150-300	qd	
Meclofenamate sodium	Meclomen	200-400	tid to qid	Higher incidence of diarrhea
Tolmetin sodium	Tolectin	800-1800	tid	Pediatric approval for JRA

Long Serum Half Life NSAIDs

Generic	Brand name	Dose Range (mg/day)*	Dose Interval	Comments
Diflunisal	Dolobid	500-1500	bid	A derivative of salicylate but not metabolized to salicylate.
Indomethacin	Indocin	50-200	bid to tid	Efficacy in ankylosing spondylitis and gout
Nabumetone	Relafen	1000-2000	qd to bid	Nonacidic pro-drug undergoes transformation to active acidic metabolite. Use with care in liver disease
Naproxen sodium	Naprosyn	750-1500	bid	Liquid available Pediatric approval for JRA
Oxaprozin	Daypro	600-1200	qd	
Piroxicam	Feldene	20	qd	
Sulindac	Clinoril	300-400	bid	May have a lower incidence of prostaglandin-mediated renal effects.

Cox-2 selective and specific NSAIDS

Generic	Brand name	Dose Range (mg/day)*	Dose Interval	Comments
Celecoxib (cox-2 specific)	Celebrex	200-400	qd to bid	No effect on platelet function. Decreased GI side effects. Contraindicated if sulfonamide allergy
Meloxicam (cox-2 selective)	Mobic	7.5 - 15	qd	No effect on platelet function. Decreased GI side effects. No adjustment for meal timing
Rofecoxib (cox-2 specific)	Vioxx	12.5-25	qd	Decreased GI side effects. Liquid available

*Doses are given as mg/day and should be divided by the dose interval when prescribing

1. Borigini, MJ and Paulus, HE. Rheumatoid Arthritis. in Weisman, MH and Weinblatt, ME. Treatment of the Rheumatic Diseases, W.B. Saunders Co.,pp 31-51, 1995
2. Physician's Desk Reference. Medical Economics Data Production Company, 2001.

11e: Medical Management of Osteoarthritis of the Hip and Knee

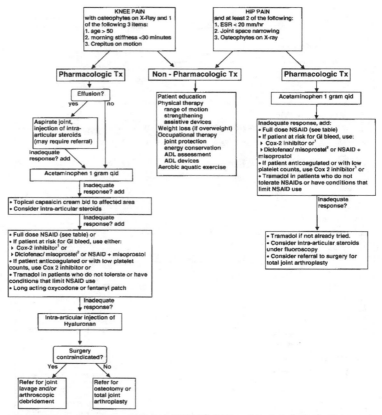

KNEE PAIN
with osteophytes on X-Ray and 1
of the following 3 items:
1. age > 50
2. morning stiffness <30 minutes
3. Crepitus on motion

HIP PAIN
and at least 2 of the following:
1. ESR < 20 mm/hr
2. Joint space narrowing
3. Osteophytes on X-ray

Pharmacologic Tx

Effusion?

yes / no

Aspirate joint,
injection of intra-
articular steroids
(may require referral)

Inadequate
response? add

Acetaminophen 1 gram qid

Inadequate
response? add

• Topical capsaicin cream bid to affected area
• Consider intra-articular steroids

Inadequate
response? add

• Full dose NSAID (see table) or
• If patient at risk for GI bleed, use either:
  ▸ Cox-2 inhibitor[1] or
  ▸ Diclofenac/ misoprostel[2] or NSAID + misoprostol
• If patient anticoagulated or with low platelet
counts, use Cox 2 inhibitor or
• Tramadol in patients who do not tolerate or have
conditions that limit NSAID use
• Long acting oxycodone or fentanyl patch

Inadequate
response?

Intra-articular injection of
Hyaluronan

Surgery
contraindicated?

Yes / No

Refer for joint
lavage and/or
arthroscopic
debridement

Refer for
osteotomy or
total joint
arthroplasty

Non - Pharmacologic Tx

Patient education
Physical therapy
  range of motion
  strengthening
  assistive devices
Weight loss (if overweight)
Occupational therapy
  joint protection
  energy conservation
  ADL assessment
  ADL devices
Aerobic aquatic exercise

Pharmacologic Tx

Acetaminophen 1 gram qid

Inadequate response, add:
• Full dose NSAID (see table)
• If patient at risk for GI bleed, use:
  ▸ Cox-2 inhibitor[1]
  ▸ Diclofenac/ misoprostel[2] or NSAID +
  misoprostol
• If patient anticoagulated or with low
platelet counts, use Cox 2 inhibitor[1] or
• Tramadol in patients who do not
tolerate NSAIDs or have conditions that
limit NSAID use

Inadequate
response?

• Tramadol if not already tried.
• Consider intra-articular steroids
under fluoroscopy
• Consider referral to surgery for
total joint arthroplasty

1. Cox-2 inhibitors: Cox-2 specific: Celecoxib 200 - 400 mg qd, Rofecoxib 12.5-25 mg qd. Cox-2 selective: Meloxicam 7.5-15 mg qd
2. misoprostol: 200 mcg qid. Use 100 mcg qid if GI symptoms occur. Tramadol: 50 – 100 mg q 4-6h
*Risk factors for GI bleed: age >75, h/o peptic ulcer disease, GI bleed, or heart disease.

Hochberg, MC. et al. Guidelines for the Medical Management of Osteoarthritis. Part I. Osteoarthritis of the Hip. Arthritis Rheum. 38:1535-1549, 1995
Hochberg, MC. et al. Guidelines for the Medical Management of Osteoarthritis. Part II. Osteoarthritis of the Knee. Arthritis Rheum. 38:1541-1546, 1995.

11f: Differential Diagnosis of Polyarthritis

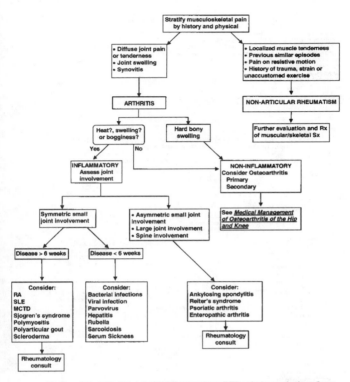

RA = rheumatoid arthritis; SLE = systemic lupus erythematosus; MCTD = mixed connective tissue disease

1. Sergent, JS. Polyarticular Arthritis. Chapter 23 in Kelley, WN. Textbook of Rheumatology. 4th Edition, W.B. Saunders Company, 381-388, 1993.
2. Pinals, RS. Polyarthritis and Fever. NEJM. 330:769-774, 1994.

11g: Medical Management of Rheumatoid Arthritis

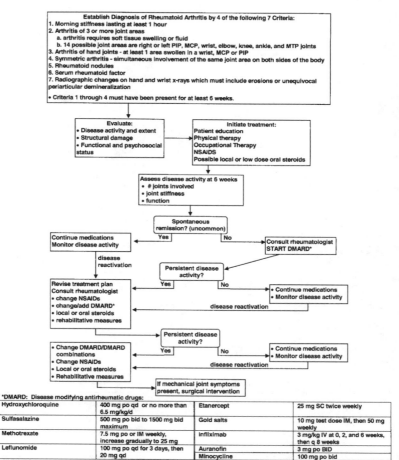

Establish Diagnosis of Rheumatoid Arthritis by 4 of the following 7 Criteria:
1. Morning stiffness lasting at least 1 hour
2. Arthritis of 3 or more joint areas
   a. arthritis requires soft tissue swelling or fluid
   b. 14 possible joint areas are right or left PIP, MCP, wrist, elbow, knee, ankle, and MTP joints
3. Arthritis of hand joints - at least 1 area swollen in a wrist, MCP or PIP
4. Symmetric arthritis - simultaneous involvement of the same joint area on both sides of the body
5. Rheumatoid nodules
6. Serum rheumatoid factor
7. Radiographic changes on hand and wrist x-rays which must include erosions or unequivocal periarticular demineralization

• Criteria 1 through 4 must have been present for at least 6 weeks.

Evaluate:
• Disease activity and extent
• Structural damage
• Functional and psychosocial status

Initiate treatment:
Patient education
Physical therapy
Occupational Therapy
NSAIDS
Possible local or low dose oral steroids

Assess disease activity at 6 weeks
• # joints involved
• joint stiffness
• function

Spontaneous remission? (uncommon)

Continue medications
Monitor disease activity — Yes

No — Consult rheumatologist START DMARD*

disease reactivation

Persistent disease activity?

Revise treatment plan
Consult rheumatologist
• change NSAIDs
• change/add DMARD*
• local or oral steroids
• rehabilitative measures

Yes

No — • Continue medications
• Monitor disease activity

disease reactivation

Persistent disease activity?

• Change DMARD/DMARD combinations
• Change NSAIDs
• Local or oral steroids
• Rehabilitative measures

Yes

No — • Continue medications
• Monitor disease activity

disease reactivation

If mechanical joint symptoms present, surgical intervention

*DMARD: Disease modifying antirheumatic drugs:

Hydroxychloroquine	400 mg po qd or no more than 6.5 mg/kg/d	Etanercept	25 mg SC twice weekly
Sulfasalazine	500 mg po bid to 1500 mg bid maximum	Gold salts	10 mg test dose IM, then 50 mg weekly
Methotrexate	7.5 mg po or IM weekly, increase gradually to 25 mg	Infliximab	3 mg/kg IV at 0, 2, and 6 weeks, then q 8 weeks
Leflunomide	100 mg po qd for 3 days, then 20 mg qd	Auranofin	3 mg po BID
		Minocycline	100 mg po bid

All DMARDs should be prescribed by physicians familiar with their use and many require specific monitoring.
1. Arnett, FC. et al. The American Rheumatism Association 1987 Revised Criteria for the Classification of Rheumatoid Arthritis. Arthritis Rheum. 31:315-324, 1988
2. American College of Rheumatology Ad Hoc Committee on Clinical Guidelines. Guidelines for the Management of Rheumatoid Arthritis. Arthritis Rheum. 39:713-722, 1996.

11h: Evaluation of Suspected Vasculitis

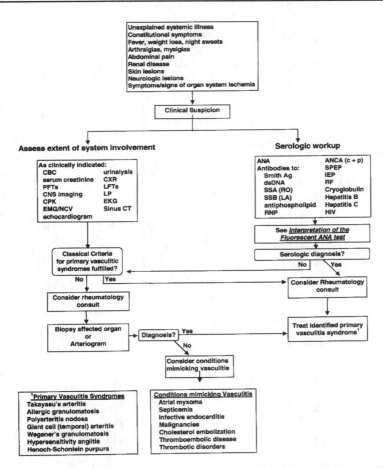

Unexplained systemic illness
Constitutional symptoms
Fever, weight loss, night sweats
Arthralgias, myalgias
Abdominal pain
Renal disease
Skin lesions
Neurologic lesions
Symptoms/signs of organ system ischemia

↓

Clinical Suspicion

Assess extent of system involvement

As clinically indicated:
CBC	urinalysis
serum creatinine	CXR
PFTs	LFTs
CNS imaging	LP
CPK	EKG
EMG/NCV	Sinus CT
echocardiogram	

Classical Criteria for primary vasculitic syndromes fulfilled?
No   Yes

Consider rheumatology consult

Biopsy affected organ or Arteriogram

Diagnosis?   Yes
No

Consider conditions mimicking vasculitis

Serologic workup

ANA	ANCA (c + p)
Antibodies to:	SPEP
Smith Ag	IEP
dsDNA	RF
SSA (RO)	Cryoglobulin
SSB (LA)	Hepatitis B
antiphospholipid	Hepatitis C
RNP	HIV

See *Interpretation of the Fluorescent ANA test*

Serologic diagnosis?
No   Yes

Consider Rheumatology consult

Treat identified primary vasculitis syndrome[1]

[1]Primary Vasculitis Syndromes
Takayasu's arteritis
Allergic granulomatosis
Polyarteritis nodosa
Giant cell (temporal) arteritis
Wegener's granulomatosis
Hypersensitivity angiitis
Henoch-Schonlein purpura

Conditions mimicking Vasculitis
Atrial myxoma
Septicemia
Infective endocarditis
Malignancies
Cholesterol embolization
Thromboembolic disease
Thrombotic disorders

ANA - antinuclear antibody. dsDNA - double stranded DNA. RNP – ribonucleoprotein. HIV-human immune deficiency virus. SPEP-serum protein electrophoresis. IEP - immune protein electrophoresis. RF - rheumatoid factor. NCV-nerve conduction velocities

Conn, DL et al. Vasculitis and Related Disorders. In Kelly WN ed, Textbook of Rheumatology, WB Saunders, pp. 1077-1102, 1993

11i: Interpretation of the Fluorescent Antinuclear Antibody Test

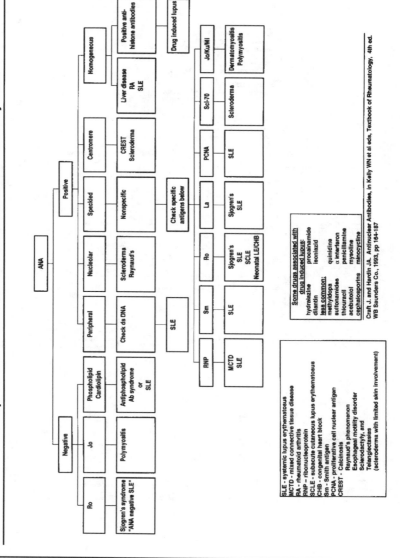

SLE - systemic lupus erythematosus
MCTD - mixed connective tissue disease
RA - rheumatoid arthritis
RNP – ribonucleoprotein
SCLE - subacute cutaneous lupus erythematosus
CHB - congenital heart block
Sm - Smith antigen
PCNA - proliferative cell nuclear antigen
CREST - Calcinosis
Raynaud's phenomenon
Esophageal motility disorder
Sclerodactyly, and
Telangiectasias
(scleroderma with limited skin involvement)

Some drugs associated with
drug induced lupus:
hydralazine   procainamide
dilantin   isoniazid
less common:
methyldopa   quinidine
sulfonamides   α interferon
thiouracil   penicillamine
acebutolol   mysoline
cephalosporins   minocycline

Craft J. and Hardin JA. Antinuclear Antibodies, in Kelly WN et al eds, Textbook of Rheumatology, 4th ed. WB Saunders Co., 1993, pp 164-187

12a: Treatment of Anaphylactic and Anaphylactoid Reactions

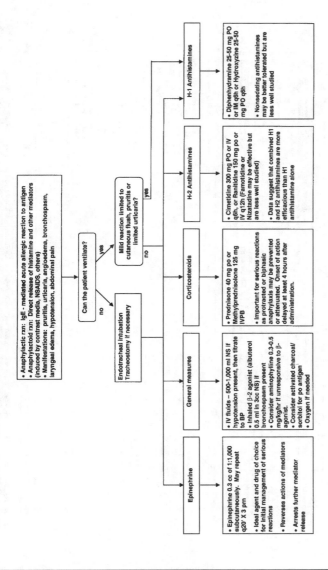

- Anaphylactic rxn: IgE - mediated acute allergic reaction to antigen
- Anaphylactoid rxn: Direct release of histamine and other mediators (induced by contrast media, NSAIDS, others)
- Manifestations: pruritis, urticaria, angioedema, bronchospasm, laryngeal edema, hypotension, abdominal pain

Can the patient ventilate?

no → Endotracheal Intubation Tracheostomy if necessary

yes → **Mild reaction limited to cutaneous flush, pruritis or limited urticaria?**

Epinephrine
- Epinephrine 0.3 cc of 1:1,000 subcutaneously. May repeat q20' X 3 prn
- Ideal agent and drug of choice for initial management of serious reactions
- Reverses actions of mediators
- Arrests further mediator release

General measures
- IV fluids – 500-1,000 ml NS if hypotension present, then titrate to BP
- Inhaled β-2 agonist (albuterol 0.5 ml in 3cc NS) if bronchospasm present
- Consider aminophylline 0.3-0.5 mg/kg/hr if unresponsive to β-agonist.
- Consider activated charcoal/ sorbitol for po antigen
- Oxygen if needed

Corticosteroids
- Prednisone 40 mg po or Methylprednisolone 125 mg IVPB
- Important for serious reactions as protracted or biphasic anaphylaxis may be prevented or attenuated. Onset of action delayed at least 4 hours after administration.

no / yes

H-2 Antihistamines
- Cimetidine 300 mg PO or IV q6h, or Ranitidine 150 mg po or IV q12h (Famotidine or Nizatadine may be effective but are less well studied)
- Data suggest that combined H1 and H2 antihistamines are more efficacious than H1 antihistamine alone

H-1 Antihistamines
- Diphenhydramine 25-50 mg PO or IM q6h or Hydroxyzine 25-50 mg PO q6h
- Nonsedating antihistamines may be better tolerated but are less well studied

Bochner BS, Lichtenstein LM. Anaphylaxis. N Engl J Med 324: 1785-1790, 1991
Stark BJ, Sullivan TJ. Biphasic and protracted anaphylaxis. J Allergy Clin Immunol 78: 76-83, 1986
Lang DM. Anaphylactoid and anaphylactic reactions: Hazards of β-adrenergic blockers. Drug Safety 12: 299-304, 1995

12b: Insect Stings: Management and Prevention of Anaphylactic Reactions from Hymenoptera Venom

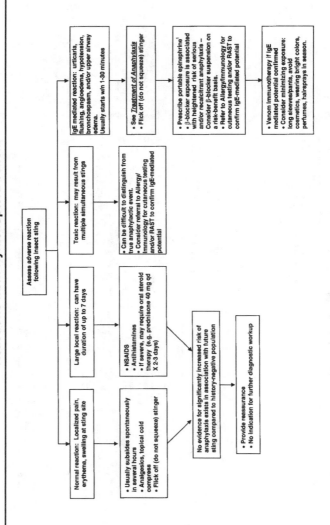

Assess adverse reaction following insect sting

Normal reaction: Localized pain, erythema, swelling at sting site
- Usually subsides spontaneously in several hours
- Analgesics, topical cold compress
- Flick off (do not squeeze) stinger

Large local reaction: can have duration of up to 7 days
- NSAIDS
- Antihistamines
- If severe, may require oral steroid therapy (e.g. prednisone 40 mg qd X 2-3 days)

No evidence for significantly increased risk of future anaphylaxis exists in association with history-negative population
- Provide reassurance
- No indication for further diagnostic workup

Toxic reaction: may result from multiple simultaneous stings
- Can be difficult to distinguish from true anaphylactic event.
- Consider referral to Allergy/Immunology for cutaneous testing and/or RAST to confirm IgE-mediated potential

IgE mediated reaction: urticaria, flushing, angioedema, hypotension, bronchospasm, and/or upper airway edema.
Usually starts w/n 1-30 minutes
- See *Treatment of Anaphylaxis*
- Flick off (do not squeeze) stinger

- Prescribe portable epinephrine[1]
- β-blocker exposure is associated with heightened risk of serious and/or recalcitrant anaphylaxis – Consider β-blocker suspension on a risk-benefit basis.
- Refer to Allergy/Immunology for cutaneous testing and/or RAST to confirm IgE-mediated potential

- Venom immunotherapy if IgE mediated potential confirmed
- Consider minimizing exposure: long sleeves/pants, avoid cosmetics, wearing bright colors, perfumes, hairsprays in season.

Portable epinephrine: 0.3 ml of 1:1,000 epinephrine (EpiPen, ANA-Kit, ANA-guard -- also contains 2 mg tablets of chlorpheniramine maleate)
Hymenoptera: Honeybees, Vespids (yellow jacket, hornet), wasp

Golden DBK, Marsh DG, Kagey-Sobotka A, Friedhoff L, Szklo M, Valentine MD, Lichtenstein LM. Epidemiology of insect venom sensitivity. JAMA 262: 240-244, 1989
Valentine MD. Allergy to stinging insects. Ann Allergy 70: 427-432, 1993
Levine MI, Lockey RF. Monograph on Insect Allergy (3rd Edition). American Acadamy of Allergy and Immunology, Dave Lambert Associates, Pittsburgh, PA, 1995.

12c: Prevention of Anaphylactoid Reactions from Intravenous Contrast Media[1]

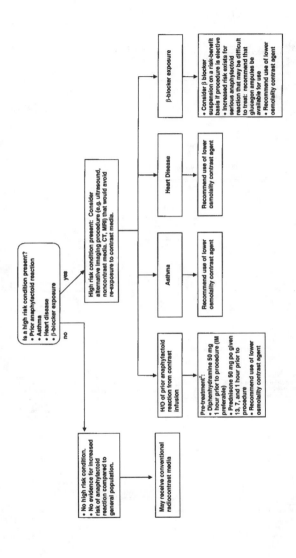

1. This does not include prevention of risk for non-anaphylactoid reactions from radiocontrast media, e.g. hemodynamic, nephrotoxicity, pulmonary edema, or other untoward reactions.
2. Pretreatment with/without use of low osmolal contrast agent reduces (but does not eliminate) risk for anaphylactoid reaction.

Greenberger PA, Patterson R, Tapio CM. Prophylaxis against repeated radiocontrast media reactions in 857 cases. Arch Intern Med 145: 2197-2200, 1985
Jacobson PD, Rosenquist J. The introduction of low-osmolar contrast agents in radiology: medical, economic, legal and public policy issues. JAMA 260: 1586-1592, 1988
Katayama H, Yagamuchi K, et al. Adverse reactions to ionic and nonionic contrast media. Radiology 175: 621-628, 1990
Lang DM, Alpern MB, Visintainer PF, Smith ST. Elevated risk for anaphylactoid reaction from radiographic contrast media is associated with both β-adrenergic blocker exposure and
  cardiovascular disorders. Arch Intern Med 153: 2033-2040, 1993
Lieberman P. Anaphylactoid reactions to radiocontrast material. Immunol Allergy Clin NA 12: 649-670, 1992
Manual on Iodinated Contrast Material. American College of Radiology, 1990

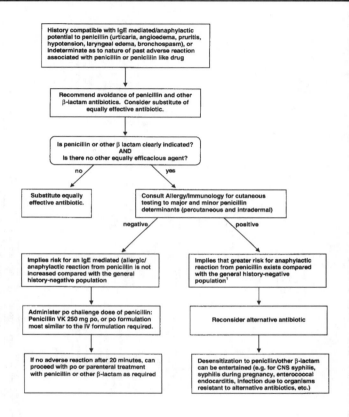

History compatible with IgE mediated/anaphylactic potential to penicillin (urticaria, angioedema, pruritis, hypotension, laryngeal edema, bronchospasm), or indeterminate as to nature of past adverse reaction associated with penicillin or penicillin like drug

Recommend avoidance of penicillin and other β-lactam antibiotics. Consider substitute of equally effective antibiotic.

Is penicillin or other β lactam clearly indicated? AND Is there no other equally efficacious agent?

no / yes

Substitute equally effective antibiotic.

Consult Allergy/Immunology for cutaneous testing to major and minor penicillin determinants (percutaneous and intradermal)

negative / positive

Implies risk for an IgE mediated (allergic/anaphylactic reaction from penicillin is not increased compared with the general history-negative population

Implies that greater risk for anaphylactic reaction from penicillin exists compared with the general history-negative population[1]

Administer po challenge dose of penicillin: Penicillin VK 250 mg po, or po formulation most similar to the IV formulation required.

Reconsider alternative antibiotic

If no adverse reaction after 20 minutes, can proceed with po or parenteral treatment with penicillin or other β-lactam as required

Desensitization to penicillin/other β-lactam can be entertained (e.g. for CNS syphilis, syphilis during pregnancy, enterococcal endocarditis, infection due to organisms resistant to alternative antibiotics, etc.)

1. Administration of other β-lactams, including carbopenims and cephalosporins may entail greater risk of anaphylaxis in penicillin allergic patients. For this reason, administration of other β-lactams should also be avoided if possible.

Saxon A, Beall GN, Rohr AS, Adelman DC. Immediate hypersensitivity reactions to β-lactam antibiotics. Ann Intern Med 107: 204-215, 1987

Sogn DD, Evans R, Shepherd GM et al. National Institute of Allergy and Infectious Diseases, Bethesda MD and other centers: Results of the National Institute of Allergy and Infectious Diseases collaborative clinical trial to test the predictive value of skin testing with major and minor penicillin derivatives in hospitalized adults. Arch Intern Med 152: 1025-1032, 1992

12e: Nasal Miseries

Diagnosis	Allergic rhinitis (AR)	NARES[1]	Nasal polyps	Vasomotor rhinitis	Chronic Sinusitis	Rhinitis Medicamentosa
Symptoms	Pruritis, congestion, clear discharge, sneezing	Clear discharge; ± pruritis	Congestion, clear discharge, *usually unilateral*	Severe congestion with copious clear discharge	Cough, URI symptoms	Congestion and rhinorrhea
Occurrence	Seasonal or perennial	Perennial	Perennial	Perennial	Perennial	Perennial
Onset	Any age	Adult	Usually adult	Adult	Any age	Any age
Associated Factors	Asthma, allergic conjunctivitis	Asthma, aspirin sensitivity	Asthma, aspirin sensitivity, allergic rhinitis (AR), cystic fibrosis, sinusitis	Women > men, sx increase with environmental and physical factors (temperature, ETOH, humidity, stress, strong odor, spicy foods)	Possible structural abnormalities, post viral URI, AR, rarely tumors	History of chronic topical decongestant use, oral antihypertensives, psychotropic drugs, or oral birth control pills
Nasal mucosa	Pale/Blue	Pale/Blue	Pale/blue gelatinous ("bag of jelly")	Edema	Red with edema	Bright red with edema
Nasal smear	Eosinophils	Eosinophils	Eosinophils	Normal	PMNs	Normal
Skin test	Positive	Negative	Negative unless associated with AR	Negative unless associated with AR	Negative unless associated with AR	Negative
Etiology	IgE-mediated	Unknown	Unknown – outpouching of lining of sinuses	Possibly autonomic dysfunction	Bacterial infection	Tachyphylaxis to topical decongestants with "rebound" congestion and rhinorrhea
Treatment	Avoidance, oral antihistamines, nasal steroids, nasal ipratropium bromide	Nasal steroids, nasal ipratropium bromide	Nasal steroids, treatment of AR or sinusitis if present, surgery if Rx fails.	Nasal steroids, oral decongestants, nasal ipratropium bromide	Antibiotics[3], nasal or oral decongestants, nasal ipratropium bromide	Stop offending medication[2]; nasal ± oral steroids, nasal ipratropium bromide

Oral nonsedating antihistamines: Cetirizine10 mg qd, Fexofenadine 60 mg bid (30 mg bid for children) or 180 mg qd, or Loratadine 10 mg qd. 1st generation antihistamines may be equally effective and are less expensive.

Nasal steroids: Beclomethasone 1 puff in each nostril bid-qid, Budesonide 2 sprays in each nostril bid, Mometasone 2 sprays in each nostril qd, Flunisolide 2 sprays in each nostril bid, Fluticasone 1-2 puffs in each nostril qd or bid, or Triamcinolone 1-2 sprays in each nostril qd

Ipratropium bromide 0.03%: 2 puffs in each nostril bid-tid for above indications. Ipratropium bromide 0.06%: 2 puffs in each nostril tid - qid X 4 days for common cold.

Oral decongestants: Pseudoephedrine 120 mg sustained release q12h; many preparations contain guaifenesin.

Mucus thinning agent: Guaifenesin 400-1200 mg bid

1. NARES – nonallergic rhinitis with eosinophilia syndrome
2. If topical agent, consider withdrawing medication one nostril at a time
3. Antibiotics: Amoxicillin/clavulinic acid 875 mg bid, trimethoprim/sulfasoxazole 1 DS BID, or cefuroxime axetil 250 mg bid for 3 weeks depending on chronicity

Metzger EO. Anticholinergic therapy for allergic and nonallergic rhinitis and the common cold. J All Clin Immunol 95(5 pt 2) May 1995
Naclerio R, Solomon W. Rhinitis and inhalant allergens. JAMA 1997 Dec 10;278(22):1842-8
Slavin RG Nasal polyps and sinusitis JAMA 1997 Dec 10;278(22):1849-54

12f: Diagnostic Workup of Recurrent Infections

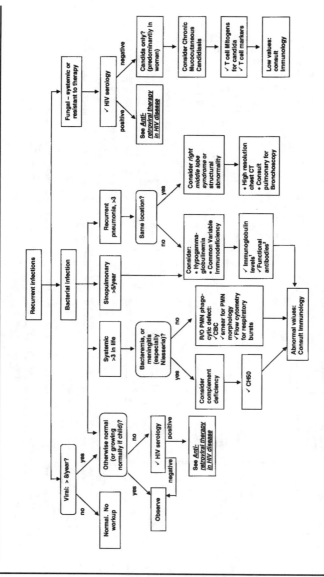

Stiehm ER. New and old immunodeficiencies. Pediatr Res (33 suppl): S2-S8, 1993
Johnson RB Jr. Recurrent bacterial infections in children. N Engl J Med 310:237-243, 1984

1. Immunoglobulin eletrophoresis and quantitative IgA, IgG, IgM, and IgG subclass levels
2. Antibodies vs. tetanus, pneumococcus, and/or H influenza. If negative, confirm by giving pneumococcal vaccine and look for response. Lack of response is c/w B-cell defect and Immunology should be consulted.

13a: Management of Diabetic Ketoacidosis

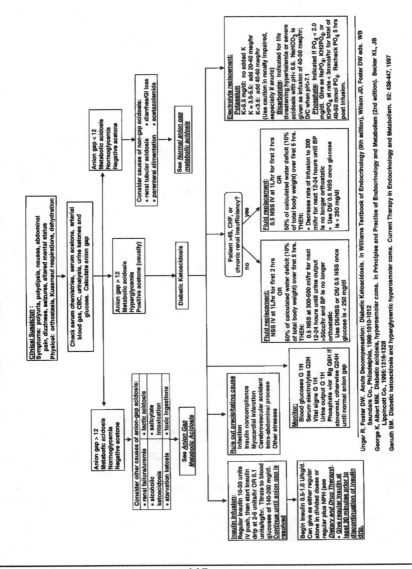

Clinical Suspicion :
Symptoms: polyuria, polydipsia, nausea, abdominal pain, dizziness, seizures, altered mental status
Physical: orthostasis, Kussmaul respirations, dehydration

Check serum chemistries, serum acetone, arterial blood gas, CBC, urinalysis, urine ketones and glucose. Calculate anion gap

Anion gap > 12
Metabolic acidosis
Normoglycemia
Negative acetone

Anion gap > 12
Metabolic acidosis
Hyperglycemia
Positive acetone (usually)

Anion gap < 12
Metabolic acidosis
Normoglycemia
Negative acetone

Consider other causes of anion-gap acidosis:
• renal failure/uremia   • lactic acidosis
• alcoholic   • salicylate
  ketoacidosis   intoxication
• starvation ketosis   • toxic ingestions

See *Anion Gap Metabolic Acidosis*

Consider causes of non-gap acidosis:
• renal tubular acidosis   • diarrhea/GI loss
• parenteral alimentation   • acetazolamide

See *Normal anion gap metabolic acidosis*

Diabetic Ketoacidosis

Insulin Infusion:
Regular insulin 10-30 units IV push, then start insulin drip at 2-5 units/hr OR 0.1 units/kg/hr. Titrate to blood glucoses of 140-200 mg/dl. Continue until anion gap is resolved

Begin insulin 0.5-1.0 U/kg/d. Can give as either regular alone in divided doses or regular plus NPH (see *Dietary and Drug Therapy*).
• Give regular insulin at least 30 minutes prior to discontinuation of insulin drip.

Rule out precipitating cause
Infection
Insulin noncompliance
Myocardial infarction
Cerebrovascular accident
Intra-abdominal process
Other stresses

Monitor:
Blood glucoses Q1H
Serum electrolytes Q2H
Vital signs Q1H
Urine output Q1H
Phosphate +/or Mg Q6H if abnormal, otherwise Q24H until normal anion gap

Patient >65, CHF, or chronic renal insufficiency?

no

Fluid replacement:
NSS IV at 1L/hr for first 2 hrs
OR
50% of calculated water deficit (10% of total body weight) over first 5 hrs.
THEN:
0.5 NSS at 300-600 ml/hr for next 12-24 hours until urine output >50cc/hr and BP is no longer orthostatic
Use D5/NSS or D5/0.5 NSS once glucose is < 250 mg/dl

yes

Fluid replacement:
0.5 NSS IV at 1L/hr for first 2 hrs
OR
50% of calculated water deficit (10% of total body weight) over first 5 hrs.
THEN:
• Decrease rate of infusion to 300 ml/hr for next 12-24 hours until BP is no longer orthostatic
• Use D5/ 0.5 NSS once glucose is < 250 mg/dl

Electrolyte replacement:
Potassium
K>5.5 mg/dl: no added K
K = 3.5-5.5: add 20-40 meq/hr
K<3.5: add 40-60 meq/hr
(Use caution in renally impaired, especially if anuric)
Bicarbonate: Indicated for life threatening hyperkalemia or severe acidosis with pH< 6.9. NaHCO₃ is given as infusion of 40-50 meq/hr; D/C when pH>7.1
Phosphate: Indicated if PO₄ < 2.0 mg/dl. Give as NaPO₄, KH2PO₄, or KHPO₄ at rate < 3mmol/hr for total of 40-50 mmol PO₄. Recheck PO₄ 5 hrs post infusion.

Unger R, Foster DW. Acute Decompensation: Diabetic Ketoacidosis. In Williams Textbook of Endocrinology (9th edition), Wilson JD, Foster DW eds. WB Saunders Co., Philadelphia, 1998:1010-1012.
George K, Albert MM. Diabetic acidosis, hyperosmolar comas. In Principles and Practice of Endocrinology and Metabolism (2nd edition), Becker KL, JB Lippincott Co., 1995:1316-1328
Genuth SM. Diabetic ketoacidosis and hyperglycemic hyperosmolar coma. Current Therapy in Endocrinology and Metabolism. 62: 438-447, 1997

13b: Management of Diabetes Mellitus

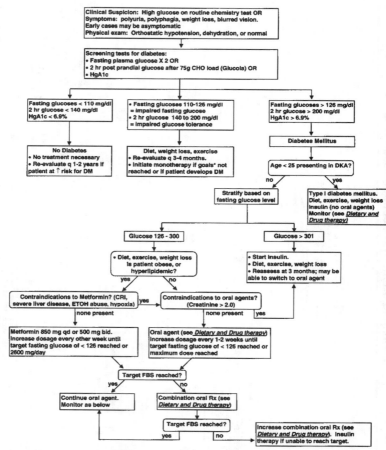

Clinical Suspicion: High glucose on routine chemistry test OR
Symptoms: polyuria, polyphagia, weight loss, blurred vision.
Early cases may be asymptomatic
Physical exam: Orthostatic hypotension, dehydration, or normal

Screening tests for diabetes:
• Fasting plasma glucose X 2 OR
• 2 hr post prandial glucose after 75g CHO load (Glucola) OR
• HgA1c

Fasting glucoses < 110 mg/dl
2 hr glucose < 140 mg/dl
HgA1c < 6.9%

• Fasting glucoses 110-126 mg/dl
= impaired fasting glucose
• 2 hr glucose 140 to 200 mg/dl
= impaired glucose tolerance

Fasting glucoses > 126 mg/dl
2 hr glucose > 200 mg/dl
HgA1c > 6.9%

No Diabetes
• No treatment necessary
• Re-evaluate q 1-2 years if
patient at ↑ risk for DM

Diet, weight loss, exercise
• Re-evaluate q 3-4 months.
• Initiate monotherapy if goals* not
reached or if patient develops DM

Diabetes Mellitus

Age < 25 presenting in DKA?

no   yes

Stratify based on
fasting glucose level

Type I diabetes mellitus.
Diet, exercise, weight loss
Insulin (no oral agents)
Monitor (see *Dietary and
Drug therapy*)

Glucose 126 - 300

Glucose > 301

• Diet, exercise, weight loss
Is patient obese, or
hyperlipidemic?

yes   no

• Start insulin.
• Diet, exercise, weight loss
• Reassess at 3 months; may be
able to switch to oral agent

Contraindications to Metformin? (CRI,
severe liver disease, ETOH abuse, hypoxia)   yes

none present

Contraindications to oral agents?
(Creatinine > 2.0)

none present   yes

Metformin 850 mg qd or 500 mg bid.
Increase dosage every other week until
target fasting glucose of < 126 reached or
2600 mg/day

Oral agent (see *Dietary and Drug therapy*)
Increase dosage every 1-2 weeks until
target fasting glucose of < 126 reached or
maximum dose reached

Target FBS reached?

yes   no

Continue oral agent.
Monitor as below

Combination oral Rx (see
Dietary and Drug therapy)

Target FBS reached?

yes   no

Increase combination oral Rx (see
Dietary and Drug therapy). Insulin
therapy if unable to reach target.

Glucose in mg/dl. BG – blood glucose, CRI – chronic renal insufficiency. FBS - fasting blood glucose. HgA1c - hemoglobin A1c. DM diabetes
mellitus.
*Goals of therapy: HbA1c < 7%, FBS 80-126, 2 hr post-prandial < 140, may add 2nd or 3rd oral agents to reach goals if no contraindication. See
Dietary and Drug Therapy for doses and contraindications.

Report of the expert committee on the diagnosis and classification of diabetes mellitus. Diabetes Care 21 (Suppl 1) S5-20, 1998
American Diabetes Association. Medical Management in NIDDM (Type II). 3rd ed, Alexandria, VA: American Diabetes Association. 1994
Edelman H. Diagnosis and management of type 2 diabetes, 3rd ed, 1999
DeFronzo RA. Pharmacologic therapy for type 2 diabetes. Ann Int Med 131 (4): 281-303. 1999

Diet: ADA (60% CHO, 20% PRO, 20% FAT); add HS snack if on oral hypoglycemic. Add 3 pm + HS snacks if pt on intermediate or long acting insulin (NPH, Lente, Ultralente)

Insulin therapy:
Types of insulin:
1. Short acting: Regular, Humalog
2. Intermediate acting: NPH, Lente
3. Long acting: Ultra Lente

- Starting dose = 0.5-1.0 units/kg/day
- 2/3 given 30' before breakfast: 1/3 short acting, 2/3 intermediate or long acting
- 1/3 given 30' before supper: 1/3 short acting, 2/3 intermediate or long acting
- Insulin must be further adjusted based on patient home monitored blood glucose.

Target blood glucoses:
- AC 80 – 120
- HS 100 – 140
- HgbA1c < 7%

Monitoring:

• Initial home glucose monitoring [before meals (AC) and before sleep (HS)] if taking insulin	• PE with neurologic exam, peripheral pulses Q3 months
• HgA1c Q 3 mos	• FBS TIW X 3 weeks for Type 2 diabetes
• Eye exam (retinopathy) Q 12 mos	• EKG, stress test for clinical indications
• Serum creatinine, 24 hr urine for microalbuminuria + creatinine clearance Q 12 mos	

Oral Agents:
- Sulfonylureas

Agent	Initial dose	Maximum dose	Contraindications
Glipizide (Glucotrol)	2.5 - 5 mg QD	40 mg po in divided doses	Renal insufficiency (creatinine > 2.0) due to risk of severe, prolonged hypoglycemia
Glipizide long acting (Glucotrol XL)	2.5 - 5 mg QD	20 mg daily	
Glyburide (Diabeta, Micronase)	1.25 2.5 mg QD	20 mg in divided doses	
Glimepiride (Amaryl)	1-2 mg qd	8 mg qd	
Micronized glyburide (Glynase PT)	1.5 – 3.0 mg qd	12 mg qd	

- Glitazones

Agent	Initial dose	Maximum dose	Contraindications
Rosiglitazone (Avandia)	2-4 mg qd	8 mg qd	↑ LFTs, ETOH abuse Class III and IV congestive heart failure (note: monitor LFTs)
Pioglitazone (Actos)	15 – 30 mg qd	45 mg qd	

- Meglitidine

Repaglinide (Prandin)	0.5 mg tid – qid before meals	4 mg po tid – qid before meals	Renal insufficiency

- Biguanide

Agent	Initial dose	Maximum dose	Contraindications
Metformin (Glucophage)	500 mg bid	2,500 mg/d	Renal insufficiency (♂ creat > 1.5, ♀ creat > 1.4), ETOH abuse, CHF, hypoxia, severe liver disease
Glucophage XR	500 mg qd		

- Alpha-glucosidase inhibitors

Agent	Initial dose	Maximum dose	Contraindications
Acarbose (Precose) Miglitol (Glycer)	25 mg tid with meals	100 mg tid with meals	↑ LFTs

Combinations may be used if needed for better glucose control. Frequently used combinations are:

1. Glyburide/metformin 2.5/500 mg and 5/500 mg (Glucovance) qd or q12h	
2. Sulfonylurea + metformin	5. Biguanide + meglitidine
3.. Sulfonylurea + glitazone	7. Sulfonylurea + biguanide + glitazone
4. Sulfonylurea + alpha-glucosidase inhibitor	8. Meglitidine + biguanide + glitazone
5. Biguanide + glitazone	9. Biguanide or glitazone + insulin

www.aace.com/clinguideindex.htm

13d: Management of Hypothyroidism

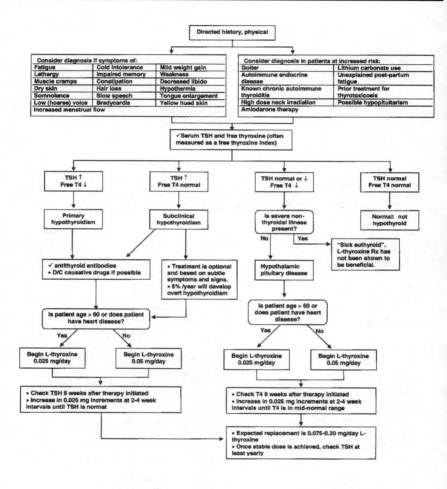

Directed history, physical

Consider diagnosis if symptoms of:

Fatigue	Cold intolerance	Mild weight gain
Lethargy	Impaired memory	Weakness
Muscle cramps	Constipation	Decreased libido
Dry skin	Hair loss	Hypothermia
Somnolence	Slow speech	Tongue enlargement
Low (hoarse) voice	Bradycardia	Yellow hued skin
Increased menstrual flow		

Consider diagnosis in patients at increased risk:

Goiter	Lithium carbonate use
Autoimmune endocrine disease	Unexplained post-partum fatigue
Known chronic autoimmune thyroiditis	Prior treatment for thyrotoxicosis
High dose neck irradiation	Possible hypopituitarism
Amiodarone therapy	

✓ Serum TSH and free thyroxine (often measured as a free thyroxine index)

TSH ↑ / Free T4 ↓
→ Primary hypothyroidism
→ ✓ antithyroid antibodies • D/C causative drugs if possible
→ Is patient age > 60 or does patient have heart disease?
- Yes → Begin L-thyroxine 0.025 mg/day
- No → Begin L-thyroxine 0.05 mg/day
→ • Check TSH 8 weeks after therapy initiated • Increase in 0.025 mg increments at 2-4 week intervals until TSH is normal

TSH ↑ / Free T4 normal
→ Subclinical hypothyroidism
→ • Treatment is optional and based on subtle symptoms and signs. • 5% /year will develop overt hypothyroidism

TSH normal or ↓ / Free T4 ↓
→ Is severe non-thyroidal illness present?
- No → Hypothalamic pituitary disease
- Yes → "Sick euthyroid". L-thyroxine Rx has not been shown to be beneficial.
→ Is patient age > 60 or does patient have heart disease?
- Yes → Begin L-thyroxine 0.025 mg/day
- No → Begin L-thyroxine 0.05 mg/day
→ • Check T4 8 weeks after therapy initiated • Increase in 0.025 mg increments at 2-4 week intervals until T4 is in mid-normal range

TSH normal / Free T4 normal
→ Normal: not hypothyroid

• Expected replacement is 0.075-0.20 mg/day L-thyroxine
• Once stable dose is achieved, check TSH at least yearly

13e: Management of Thyrotoxicosis

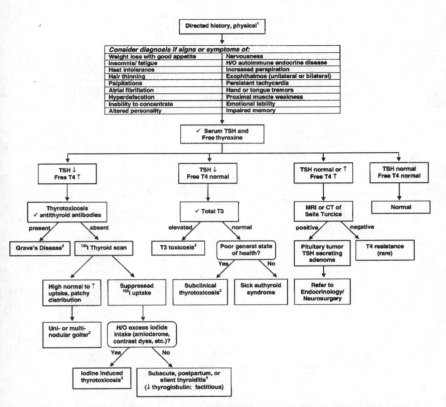

Directed history, physical[1]

Consider diagnosis if signs or symptoms of:

Weight loss with good appetite	Nervousness
Insomnia/ fatigue	H/O autoimmune endocrine disease
Heat intolerance	Increased perspiration
Hair thinning	Exophthalmos (unilateral or bilateral)
Palpitations	Persistent tachycardia
Atrial fibrillation	Hand or tongue tremors
Hyperdefecation	Proximal muscle weakness
Inability to concentrate	Emotional lability
Altered personality	Impaired memory

✓ Serum TSH and Free thyroxine

- **TSH ↓ Free T4 ↑**
  - Thyrotoxicosis ✓ antithyroid antibodies
    - **present** → Grave's Disease[2]
    - **absent** → ¹²³I Thyroid scan
      - High normal to ↑ uptake, patchy distribution → Uni- or multi-nodular goiter[2]
      - Suppressed ¹²³I uptake → H/O excess iodide intake (amiodarone, contrast dyes, etc.)?
        - **Yes** → Iodine induced thyrotoxicosis[3]
        - **No** → Subacute, postpartum, or silent thyroiditis[4] (↓ thyroglobulin: factitious)

- **TSH ↓ Free T4 normal**
  - ✓ Total T3
    - **elevated** → T3 toxicosis[2]
    - **normal** → Poor general state of health?
      - **Yes** → Subclinical thyrotoxicosis[2]
      - **No** → Sick euthyroid syndrome

- **TSH normal or ↑ Free T4 ↑**
  - MRI or CT of Sella Turcica
    - **positive** → Pituitary tumor TSH secreting adenoma → Refer to Endocrinology/ Neurosurgery
    - **negative** → T4 resistance (rare)

- **TSH normal Free T4 normal**
  - Normal

1. Grave's disease goiters are generally smooth. Multinodular goiters have nodules of different sizes. Uninodular glands have a solitary nodule, which may consume much of a lobe. Subacute thyroiditis often presents with viral prodrome, persistent neck tenderness and sore throat. The ESR is increased. Postpartum thyroiditis may present with thyrotoxicosis or hypothyroidism.
2. Treat with propylthiouracil (PTU, start at 100 mg TID) or methimazole (start at 10-30 mg QD) until T4 levels depleted (1 to several months). β-blockers for symptomatic relief. Refer to Endocrinology for ¹³¹I ablation (contraindicated in pregnancy; many avoid use of ¹³¹I in children and fertile women; higher doses required for nodular goiter). Surgical excision is an option for Graves' disease and resistant nodules. Monitor for hypothyroidism after treatment.
3. Treat with PTU or methimazole plus β-blockers until thyroidal iodine is depleted. If amiodarone is required, antithyroid drugs can be continued.
4. Usually self limited. β-blockers useful for symptomatic relief of thyrotoxicosis. ASA for neck tenderness. For severe thyrotoxicosis or pain, may use prednisone 40-60 mg/day, taper over 7-10 days. Selected patients benefit from continued prednisone 10 mg/d until normal ¹²³I uptake is restored.
Note: In severe recalcitrant thyrotoxicosis in the medically unstable patient, high dose PTU (600-1000mg/d), ipodate sodium (0.5 g/d), and prednisone 60 mg/d can be given until surgical resection of the thyroid can be safely undertaken

13f: Adrenal Insufficiency

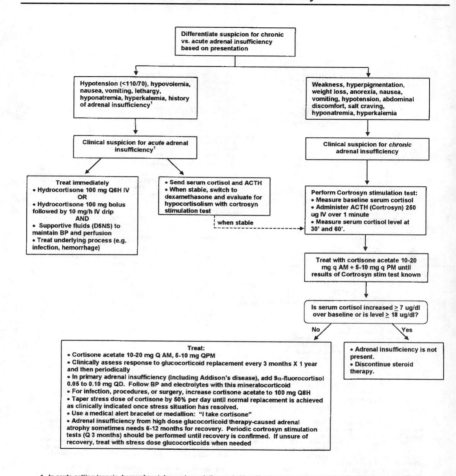

1. In acute setting (sepsis, hemorrhage), hyperpigmentation probably will not accompany metabolic effects of hypoadrenalism. In sudden glucocorticoid withdrawal in patients on chronic glucocorticoid therapy, aldosterone is intact and K+ is normal.

13g: Cushing's Syndrome

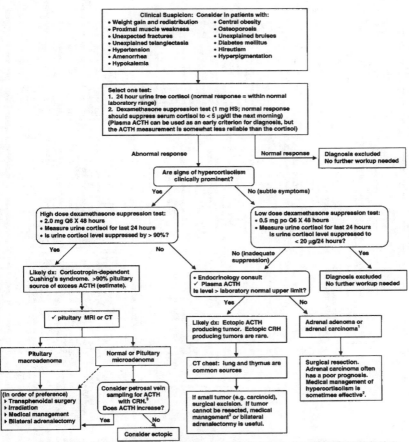

Clinical Suspicion: Consider in patients with:
- Weight gain and redistribution
- Proximal muscle weakness
- Unexpected fractures
- Unexplained telangiectasia
- Hypertension
- Amenorrhea
- Hypokalemia
- Central obesity
- Osteoporosis
- Unexplained bruises
- Diabetes mellitus
- Hirsutism
- Hyperpigmentation

↓

Select one test:
1. 24 hour urine free cortisol (normal response = within normal laboratory range)
2. Dexamethasone suppression test (1 mg HS; normal response should suppress serum cortisol to < 5 µg/dl the next morning) (Plasma ACTH can be used as an early criterion for diagnosis, but the ACTH measurement is somewhat less reliable than the cortisol)

Abnormal response → **Are signs of hypercortisolism clinically prominent?**

Normal response → Diagnosis excluded. No further workup needed

Are signs of hypercortisolism clinically prominent?
- **Yes** →
- **No (subtle symptoms)** →

Yes: High dose dexamethasone suppression test:
- 2.0 mg Q6 X 48 hours
- Measure urine cortisol for last 24 hours
- is urine cortisol level suppressed by > 90%?

No (subtle symptoms): Low dose dexamethasone suppression test:
- 0.5 mg po Q6 X 48 hours
- Measure urine cortisol for last 24 hours is urine cortisol level suppressed to < 20 µg/24 hours?

High dose test — **Yes**: Likely dx: Corticotropin-dependent Cushing's syndrome. >90% pituitary source of excess ACTH (estimate).

High dose test — **No** →

Low dose test — **No (inadequate suppression)** →

Low dose test — **Yes**: Diagnosis excluded. No further workup needed

✓ pituitary MRI or CT

↓ (from likely corticotropin-dependent)

Pituitary macroadenoma / **Normal or Pituitary microadenoma**

Pituitary macroadenoma:
(In order of preference)
▸ Transphenoidal surgery
▸ Irradiation
▸ Medical management
▸ Bilateral adrenalectomy

Normal or Pituitary microadenoma: Consider petrosal vein sampling for ACTH with CRH.[3] Does ACTH increase?
- **Yes** → (to surgery box)
- **No** → Consider ectopic

Endocrinology consult
✓ Plasma ACTH
Is level > laboratory normal upper limit?
- **Yes** →
- **No** →

Yes: Likely dx: Ectopic ACTH producing tumor. Ectopic CRH producing tumors are rare.

CT chest: lung and thymus are common sources

If small tumor (e.g. carcinoid), surgical excision. If tumor cannot be resected, medical management[2] or bilateral adrenalectomy is useful.

No: Adrenal adenoma or adrenal carcinoma[1]

Surgical resection. Adrenal carcinoma often has a poor prognosis. Medical management of hypercortisolism is sometimes effective[2].

CRH – corticotropin releasing hormone. May attain greater usefulness as screening test in the future. About 65% of patients with Cushing's syndrome have a pituitary source for ↑ ACTH (Cushing's disease). Rapid onset of Cushing's syndrome with hyperpigmentation and hypokalemia increase probability of ectopic ACTH source. No test for diagnosing Cushing's is absolute.
1. Adrenal adenomas are mainly cortisol producers with little or no androgens. Adrenal carcinomas are often > 5 cm and may produce a variety of hormones including adrenal androgens or may be silent.
2. Ketoconazole 600-1200 mg/d is the drug of choice but has liver toxicity. Metyrapone with aminoglutethimide or mitotane is also useful. Patients with ectopic ACTH tumors can break through medical therapy.
3. Controversial. A non-pituitary source would be rare and petrosal vein sampling is not always available. Dashed line indicates acceptable alternative

14a: Diagnosis and Treatment of Primary Headache

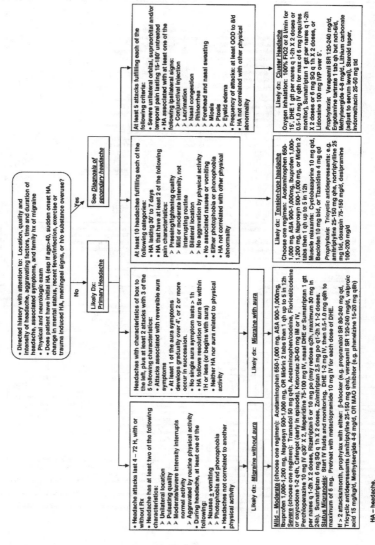

- Directed history with attention to: Location, quality and intensity of headache, aggravating factors, time and duration of headache, associated symptoms, and family hx of migraine
- Physical and neurologic exam
- Does patient have initial HA (esp if age>40, sudden onset, HA, change in mental status, recent fever/infection, exercise or trauma induced HA, meningeal signs, or h/o substance overuse?

Yes → See *Diagnosis of secondary headache*

No → Likely Dx: *Primary Headache*

- Headache attacks last 4 – 72 H, with or without fix
- Headache has at least two of the following characteristics:
  ➢ Unilateral location
  ➢ Pulsating quality
  ➢ Moderate/severe intensity interrupts normal activity
  ➢ Aggravated by routine physical activity
- During headache, at least one of the following:
  ➢ Nausea ± vomiting
  ➢ Photophobia and phonophobia
- Headaches not correlated to another physical activity

Headaches with characteristics of box to the left, plus at least 2 attacks with 3 of the 5 following characteristics:
- Attacks associated with reversible aura symptoms
- At least 1 of the aura symptoms develops gradually over 4", or 2 or more occur in succession.
- No single aura symptom lasts > 1h
- HA follows resolution of aura Sx within 1H or less (or begins with aura)
- Neither HA nor aura related to physical activity

At least 10 headaches fulfilling each of the following categories:
- HA lasting 30' to 7 days
- HA that have at least 2 of the following pain characteristics:
  ➢ Pressing/tightening quality
  ➢ Mild or moderate intensity, not interrupting routine
  ➢ Bilateral HA
  ➢ No aggravation by physical activity
- No associated nausea or vomiting
- Either photophobia or phonophobia
- HA not correlated with other physical abnormality

At least 5 attacks fulfilling each of the following criteria:
- Severe unilateral orbital, supraorbital and/or temporal pain lasting 15-180' untreated
- HA associated with at least one of the following ipsilateral signs:
  ➢ Conjunctival injection
  ➢ Lacrimation
  ➢ Nasal congestion
  ➢ Rhinorrhea
  ➢ Forehead and nasal swelling
  ➢ Miosis
  ➢ Ptosis
  ➢ Eyelid edema
- Frequency of attacks: at least QOD to 8/d
- HA not correlated with other physical abnormality

Likely dx: **Migraine without aura**

Likely dx: **Migraine with aura**

Likely dx: **Tension-type headache**

Likely dx: **Cluster Headache**

Mild – Moderate (choose one regimen): Acetaminophen 650-1,000 mg, ASA 900-1,000mg, Ibuprofen 1,000-1,200 mg, Naprosyn 500-1,000 mg, OR Midrin 2 tabs then 1 qh up to 5 in 12h
Severe (choose one regimen): Tramadol 50 mg q4h, Acetaminophen/codeine, Fioricet/codeine or oxycodone 1-2 q4h, Cafergot (early in episode), Ketorolac 30-60 mg IM or IV, Perchlorperazine 10 mg IV q30' X 2, Meperidine 75-100 mg IV, nasal DHE or Sumatriptan 1 gtt per nares q 1-2h X 2 doses, Rizatriptan 5 or 10 mg po (may redose q2h, maximum 30 mg in 24h). Sumatriptan 6 mg SQ q 1h X 2 doses, Zolmitriptan 2.5 mg po q1-2h X 1-2 doses.
Status Migrainosis: Start IV fluids and monitoring. DHE 1-2 mg IV, then 0.5-1.0 mg q8h to maximum of 6 mg. Pretreat with metaclopramide 10 mg IV for each dose of DHE.

If > 2 attacks/month, prophylax with either: β-blocker (e.g. propranolol SR 80-240 mg qd, Tricyclic antidepressants (amitriptyline 25-150 mg qhs), verapamil SR 120-240 mg/d, valproic acid 15 mg/kg/d, Methylsergide 4-8 mg/d, OR MAO inhibitor (e.g. phenelzine 15-20 mg q8h)

Likely dx: **Tension-type headache**
Choose one regimen: Acetaminophen 650-1,000 mg. ASA 900-1,000mg, Ibuprofen 650-1,200 mg, Naprosyn 500-1,000 mg, or Midrin 2 tabs then 1 qh up to 5 in 12h
Muscle relaxants: Cyclobezaprine 10 mg qid, Baclofen 10 mg bid, or Tizanidine 4 mg qd
Prophylaxis: Tricyclic antidepressants: e.g. amitriptyline 25-150 mg qhs, nortriptyline 25 mg tid, doxepin 75-150 mg/d, desipramine 100-200 mg/d

Likely dx: **Cluster Headache**
Oxygen inhalation: 100% FiO2 or 8 l/min for 15', DHE 1 gtt per nares q 1-2h X 2 doses or 0.5-1.0 mg IV q8h for max of 6 mg (requires monitor), Sumatriptan 1 gtt per nares q 1-2h X 2 doses or 6 mg SQ q 1h X 2 doses, or Lidocaine 100 mg IVP over 5'.
Prophylaxis: Verapamil SR 120-240 mg/d, Ergotamine tartrate 1 tab qh but not-6/d, Methylsergide 4-8 mg/d, Lithium carbonate (adjust to serum level), Steroid taper, Indomethacin 25-50 mg tid

---

HA – headache.
Cutrer M. Headache In Borsook D, LeBel AA, McPeak B (eds). The Massachussetts General Hospital Handbook of Pain Management. Little Brown, Boston, 1996: 270-302

122

14b: Diagnosis of Secondary Headache

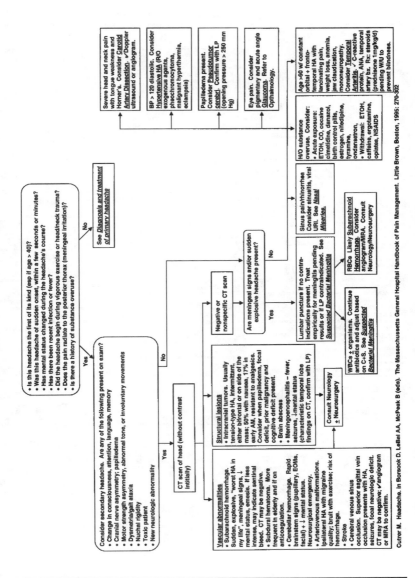

Cutter M. Headache. In Borsook D, LeBel AA, McPeak B (eds). The Massachussetts General Hospital Handbook of Pain Management. Little Brown, Boston, 1995: 270-302

123

14c: Coma and Drowsiness

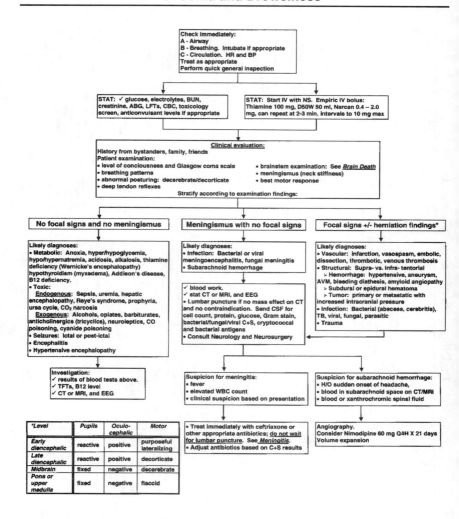

Check immediately:
A - Airway
B - Breathing. Intubate if appropriate
C - Circulation. HR and BP
Treat as appropriate
Perform quick general inspection

STAT: ✓ glucose, electrolytes, BUN, creatinine, ABG, LFTs, CBC, toxicology screen, anticonvulsant levels if appropriate

STAT: Start IV with NS. Empiric IV bolus: Thiamine 100 mg, D50W 50 ml, Narcan 0.4 – 2.0 mg, can repeat at 2-3 min. intervals to 10 mg max

Clinical evaluation:
History from bystanders, family, friends
Patient examination:
• level of conciousness and Glasgow coma scale
• breathing patterns
• abnormal posturing: decerebrate/decorticate
• deep tendon reflexes
• brainstem examination: See Brain Death
• meningismus (neck stiffness)
• best motor response
Stratify according to examination findings:

No focal signs and no meningismus

Likely diagnoses:
• Metabolic: Anoxia, hyper/hypoglycemia, hypo/hypernatremia, acidosis, alkalosis, thiamine deficiency (Wernicke's encephalopathy) hypothyroidism (myxedema), Addison's disease, B12 deficiency.
• Toxic:
  Endogenous: Sepsis, uremia, hepatic encephalopathy, Reye's syndrome, prophyria, urea cycle, CO_2 narcosis
  Exogenous: Alcohols, opiates, barbiturates, anticholinergics (tricyclics), neuroleptics, CO poisoning, cyanide poisoning
• Seizures: Ictal or post-ictal
• Encephalitis
• Hypertensive encephalopathy

Investigation:
✓ results of blood tests above.
✓ TFTs, B12 level
✓ CT or MRI, and EEG

*Level	Pupils	Oculo-cephalic	Motor
Early diencephalic	reactive	positive	purposeful lateralizing
Late diencephalic	reactive	positive	decorticate
Midbrain	fixed	negative	decerebrate
Pons or upper medulla	fixed	negative	flaccid

Meningismus with no focal signs

Likely diagnoses:
• Infection: Bacterial or viral meningoencephalitis, fungal meningitis
• Subarachnoid hemorrhage

✓ blood work.
✓ stat CT or MRI, and EEG
• Lumbar puncture if no mass effect on CT and no contraindication. Send CSF for cell count, protein, glucose, Gram stain, bacterial/fungal/viral C+S, cryptococcal and bacterial antigens
• Consult Neurology and Neurosurgery

Suspicion for meningitis:
• fever
• elevated WBC count
• clinical suspicion based on presentation

• Treat immediately with ceftriaxone or other appropriate antibiotics; do not wait for lumbar puncture. See Meningitis.
• Adjust antibiotics based on C+S results

Focal signs +/- herniation findings*

Likely diagnoses:
• Vascular: infarction, vasospasm, embolic, dissection, thrombotic, venous thrombosis
• Structural: Supra- vs. infra- tentorial
  ➢ Hemorrhage: hypertensive, aneurysm, AVM, bleeding diathesis, amyloid angiopathy
  ➢ Subdural or epidural hematoma
  increased intracranial pressure
• Infection: Bacterial (abscess, cerebritis), TB, viral, fungal, parasitic
• Trauma

Suspicion for subarachnoid hemorrhage:
• H/O sudden onset of headache,
• blood in subarachnoid space on CT/MRI
• blood or xanthrochromic spinal fluid

Angiography.
Consider Nimodipine 60 mg Q4H X 21 days
Volume expansion

14d: Status Epilepticus: Diagnostic Algorithm

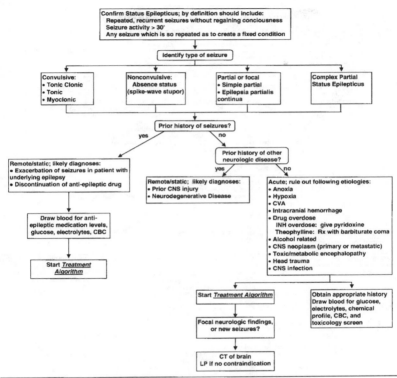

Confirm Status Epilepticus; by definition should include:
Repeated, recurrent seizures without regaining conciousness
Seizure activity > 30'
Any seizure which is so repeated as to create a fixed condition

Identify type of seizure

Convulsive:
• Tonic Clonic
• Tonic
• Myoclonic

Nonconvulsive:
Absence status
(spike-wave stupor)

Partial or focal
• Simple partial
• Epilepsia partialis continua

Complex Partial
Status Epilepticus

Prior history of seizures?
yes / no

Prior history of other neurologic disease?
yes / no

Remote/static; likely diagnoses:
• Exacerbation of seizures in patient with underlying epilepsy
• Discontinuation of anti-epileptic drug

Remote/static; likely diagnoses:
• Prior CNS injury
• Neurodegenerative Disease

Acute; rule out following etiologies:
• Anoxia
• Hypoxia
• CVA
• Intracranial hemorrhage
• Drug overdose
  INH overdose: give pyridoxine
  Theophylline: Rx with barbiturate coma
• Alcohol related
• CNS neoplasm (primary or metastatic)
• Toxic/metabolic encephalopathy
• Head trauma
• CNS infection

Draw blood for anti-epileptic medication levels, glucose, electrolytes, CBC

Start *Treatment Algorithm*

Start *Treatment Algorithm*

Obtain appropriate history
Draw blood for glucose, electrolytes, chemical profile, CBC, and toxicology screen

Focal neurologic findings, or new seizures?

CT of brain
LP if no contraindication

Urgent treatment for the most common types of status epilepticus is imperative because:
1. Prolonged (>60') seizures may be associated with neuronal injury
2. The medical problems associated with prolonged status can be severe and life threatening
3. Status epilepticus can be seen in association with other neurologic or medical emergencies (i.e. cerebral hemorrhage, CNS infection).
4. The longer status epilepticus persists, the more refractory it becomes

Sequelae of Status Epilepticus:
Most are preventable with appropriate treatment of status epilepticus and associated medical concomitants.
• Arrhythmias (patient should be monitored)
• Hyperpyrexia (usually remits when status stops)
• Rhabdomyolysis (may require saline diuresis)
• Catecholamine release
• Altered cerebral autoregulation
• Lactic acidosis
• CSF pleocytosis
• Aspiration pneumonia
• Shock (late)
• Leukocytosis
• Pulmonary edema
• Hyperkalemia
• Hypoxia

Terminating status epilepticus usually treats status-related hypertension – avoid hypotension. The agents used to treat refractory status cause hypotension and respiratory depression.

14e: Status Epilepticus: Treatment Algorithm

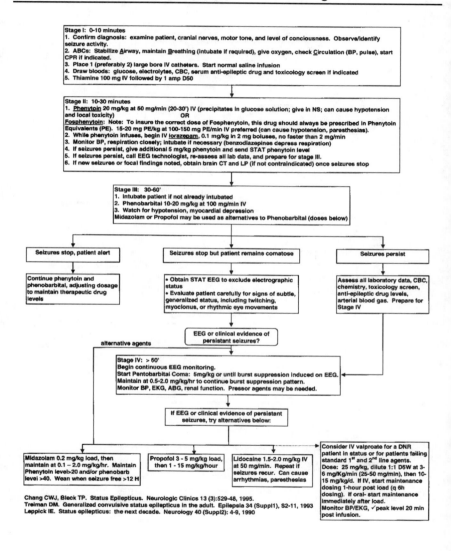

Stage I: 0-10 minutes
1. Confirm diagnosis: examine patient, cranial nerves, motor tone, and level of conciousness. Observe/identify seizure activity.
2. ABCs: Stabilize Airway, maintain Breathing (intubate if required), give oxygen, check Circulation (BP, pulse), start CPR if indicated.
3. Place 1 (preferably 2) large bore IV catheters. Start normal saline infusion
4. Draw bloods: glucose, electrolytes, CBC, serum anti-epileptic drug and toxicology screen if indicated
5. Thiamine 100 mg IV followed by 1 amp D50

Stage II: 10-30 minutes
1. Phenytoin 20 mg/kg at 50 mg/min (20-30') IV (precipitates in glucose solution; give in NS; can cause hypotension and local toxicity) OR
Fosphenytoin: Note: To insure the correct dose of Fosphenytoin, this drug should always be prescribed in Phenytoin Equivalents (PE). 15-20 mg PE/kg at 100-150 mg PE/min IV preferred (can cause hypotension, paresthesias).
2. While phenytoin infuses, begin IV lorazepam, 0.1 mg/kg in 2 mg boluses, no faster than 2 mg/min
3. Monitor BP, respiration closely; intubate if necessary (benzodiazepines depress respiration)
4. If seizures persist, give additional 5 mg/kg phenytoin and send STAT phenytoin level
5. If seizures persist, call EEG technologist, re-assess all lab data, and prepare for stage III.
6. If new seizures or focal findings noted, obtain brain CT and LP (if not contraindicated) once seizures stop

Stage III: 30-60'
1. Intubate patient if not already intubated
2. Phenobarbital 10-20 mg/kg at 100 mg/min IV
3. Watch for hypotension, myocardial depression
Midazolam or Propofol may be used as alternatives to Phenobarbital (doses below)

Seizures stop, patient alert

Continue phenytoin and phenobarbital, adjusting dosage to maintain therapeutic drug levels

Seizures stop but patient remains comatose

• Obtain STAT EEG to exclude electrographic status
• Evaluate patient carefully for signs of subtle, generalized status, including twitching, myoclonus, or rhythmic eye movements

Seizures persist

Assess all laboratory data, CBC, chemistry, toxicology screen, anti-epileptic drug levels, arterial blood gas. Prepare for Stage IV

EEG or clinical evidence of persistant seizures?

alternative agents

Stage IV: > 60'
Begin continuous EEG monitoring.
Start Pentobarbital Coma: 5mg/kg or until burst suppression induced on EEG.
Maintain at 0.5-2.0 mg/kg/hr to continue burst suppression pattern.
Monitor BP, EKG, ABG, renal function. Pressor agents may be needed.

If EEG or clinical evidence of persistant seizures, try alternatives below:

Midazolam 0.2 mg/kg load, then maintain at 0.1 – 2.0 mg/kg/hr. Maintain Phenytoin level>20 and/or phenobarb level >40. Wean when seizure free >12 H

Propofol 3 - 5 mg/kg load, then 1 - 15 mg/kg/hour

Lidocaine 1.5-2.0 mg/kg IV at 50 mg/min. Repeat if seizures recur. Can cause arrhythmias, paresthesias

Consider IV valproate for a DNR patient in status or for patients failing standard 1st and 2nd line agents. Dose: 25 mg/kg, dilute 1:1 D5W at 3-6 mg/Kg/min (25-50 mg/min), then 10-15 mg/kg/d. If IV, start maintenance dosing 1-hour post load (q 6h dosing). If oral- start maintenance immediately after load. Monitor BP/EKG, ✓peak level 20 min post infusion.

Chang CWJ, Bleck TP. Status Epilepticus. Neurologic Clinics 13 (3):529-48, 1995.
Treiman DM. Generalized convulsive status epilepticus in the adult. Epilepsia 34 (Suppl1), S2-11, 1993
Leppick IE. Status epilepticus: the next decade. Neurology 40 (Suppl2): 4-9, 1990

14f: Acute Stroke

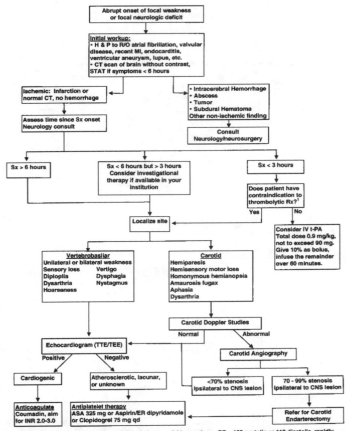

Abrupt onset of focal weakness or focal neurologic deficit

Initial workup:
• H & P to R/O atrial fibrillation, valvular disease, recent MI, endocarditis, ventricular aneurysm, lupus, etc.
• CT scan of brain without contrast, STAT if symptoms < 6 hours

Ischemic: Infarction or normal CT, no hemorrhage

• Intracerebral Hemorrhage
• Abscess
• Tumor
• Subdural Hematoma
Other non-ischemic finding

Assess time since Sx onset Neurology consult

Consult Neurology/neurosurgery

Sx > 6 hours

Sx < 6 hours but > 3 hours Consider investigational therapy if available in your institution

Sx < 3 hours

Does patient have contraindication to thrombolytic Rx?[1]
Yes / No

Consider IV t-PA Total dose 0.9 mg/kg, not to exceed 90 mg. Give 10% as bolus, infuse the remainder over 60 minutes.

Localize site

Vertebrobasilar
Unilateral or bilateral weakness
Sensory loss   Vertigo
Diplopia   Dysphagia
Dysarthria   Nystagmus
Hoarseness

Carotid
Hemiparesis
Hemisensory motor loss
Homonymous hemianopsia
Amaurosis fugax
Aphasia
Dysarthria

Carotid Doppler Studies
Normal / Abnormal

Carotid Angiography

Echocardiogram (TTE/TEE)
Positive / Negative

Cardiogenic

Atherosclerotic, lacunar, or unknown

<70% stenosis Ipsilateral to CNS lesion

70 - 99% stenosis Ipsilateral to CNS lesion

Anticoagulate Coumadin, aim for INR 2.0-3.0

Antiplatelet therapy
ASA 325 mg or Aspirin/ER dipyridamole or Clopidogrel 75 mg qd

Refer for Carotid Endarterectomy

[1]CVA or head trauma within 3 mos, major surgery within 14 days, h/o intracranial hemorrhage, BP > 185 systolic or 110 diastolic, rapidly improving or minor Sx, Sx suggestive of subarachnoid hemorrhage, GI or GU hemorrhage within 21 days, arterial puncture at a noncompressible site within 7 days, seizure at onset of stroke.

The National Institute of Neurological Disorders and Stroke rt-PA stroke study group. Tissue Plasminogen Activator for acute ischemic stroke. N Engl J Med 1995; 333:1581-1587
Chanerro A, Vica N, Saiz A, Aidery, Toiosa E. Early anticoagulation of the large cerebral infarction: a safety study. Neurology 1995; 45:861-865
Bellavane A. Efficacy of ticlopidine and aspirin for prevention of reversible cerebrovascular ischemic events: The ticlopidine aspririn stroke study. 1993; 24:1452-1457

14g: Secondary Prevention of Ischemic Stroke

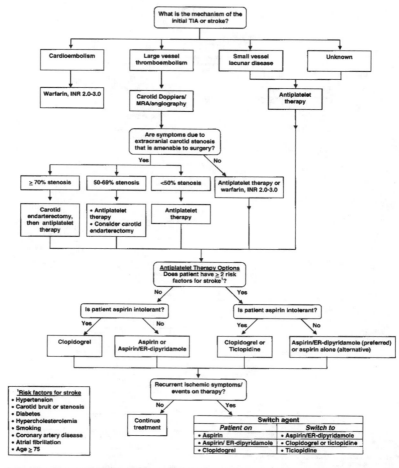

Clopidogrel: 75 mg qd. Ticlopidine: 250 mg bid (monitor CBC/platelets on ticlopidine due to risk of TTP, hematologic complications. Risk highest 1st 3 months). Aspirin: 50 to 325 mg qd. Aspirin/ER-dipyridamole: aspirin 25 mg + ER-dipyridamole 200 mg.

Fayad PB. Ischemic Cerebrovascular Disease. In Rakel RE ed. Conn's Current Therapy 1999. WB Saunders Co., Philadelphia, 885-91, 1999
Albers GW et al. Antithrombotic and Thrombolytic Therapy for Ischemic Stroke. Chest 114: 683S-98S, 1998

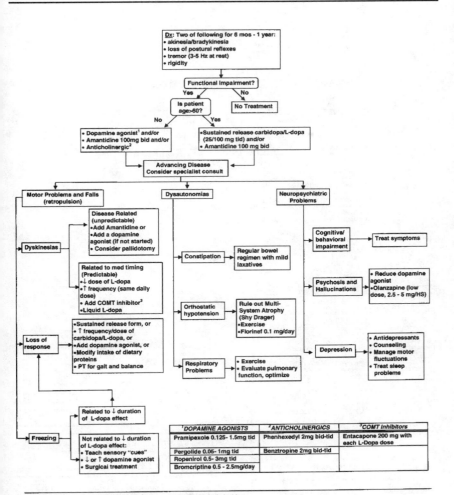

Dx: Two of following for 6 mos - 1 year:
- akinesia/bradykinesia
- loss of postural reflexes
- tremor (3-5 Hz at rest)
- rigidity

Functional Impairment?
- Yes
- No → No Treatment

Is patient age>60?
- No
- Yes

No:
- Dopamine agonist[1] and/or
- Amantidine 100mg bid and/or
- Anticholinergic[2]

Yes:
- Sustained release carbidopa/L-dopa (25/100 mg tid) and/or
- Amantidine 100 mg bid

Advancing Disease
Consider specialist consult

Motor Problems and Falls (retropulsion)

Dyskinesias:

Disease Related (unpredictable)
- Add Amantidine or
- Add a dopamine agonist (if not started)
- Consider pallidotomy

Related to med timing (Predictable)
- ↓ dose of L-dopa
- ↑ frequency (same daily dose)
- Add COMT inhibitor[3]
- Liquid L-dopa

Loss of response:
- Sustained release form, or
- ↑ frequency/dose of carbidopa/L-dopa, or
- Add dopamine agonist, or
- Modify intake of dietary proteins
- PT for gait and balance

Freezing:

Related to ↓ duration of L-dopa effect

Not related to ↓ duration of L-dopa effect:
- Teach sensory "cues"
- ↓ or ↑ dopamine agonist
- Surgical treatment

Dysautonomias

Constipation → Regular bowel regimen with mild laxatives

Orthostatic hypotension → Rule out Multi-System Atrophy (Shy Drager)
- Exercise
- Florinef 0.1 mg/day

Respiratory Problems →
- Exercise
- Evaluate pulmonary function, optimize

Neuropsychiatric Problems

Cognitive/behavioral impairment → Treat symptoms

Psychosis and Hallucinations →
- Reduce dopamine agonist
- Olanzapine (low dose, 2.5 - 5 mg/HS)

Depression →
- Antidepressants
- Counseling
- Manage motor fluctuations
- Treat sleep problems

[1]DOPAMINE AGONISTS	[2]ANTICHOLINERGICS	[3]COMT Inhibitors
Pramipexole 0.125- 1.5mg tid	Phenhexedyl 2mg bid-tid	Entacapone 200 mg with each L-Dopa dose
Pergolide 0.05- 1mg tid	Benztropine 2mg bid-tid	
Ropenirol 0.5- 3mg tid		
Bromcriptine 0.5 - 2.5mg/day		

Kurlan R. 1995.Treatment of Movement Disorders. JB Lippincott, Philadelphia

14i: Evaluation and Treatment of Suspected Bacterial Meningitis

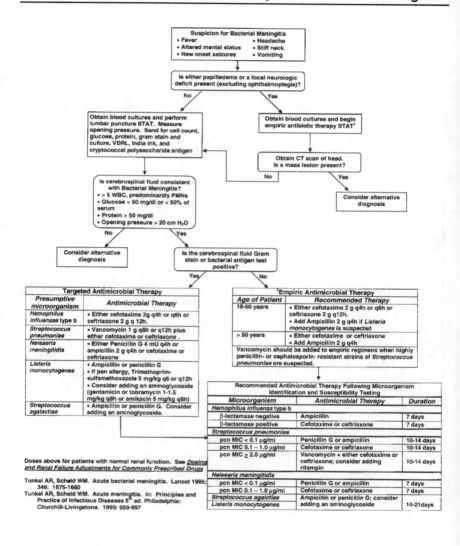

Suspicion for Bacterial Meningitis
- Fever
- Altered mental status
- New onset seizures
- Headache
- Stiff neck
- Vomiting

Is either papilledema or a focal neurologic deficit present (excluding ophthalmoplegia)?

No → Obtain blood cultures and perform lumbar puncture STAT. Measure opening pressure. Send for cell count, glucose, protein, gram stain and culture, VDRL, India ink, and cryptococcal polysaccharide antigen

Yes → Obtain blood cultures and begin empiric antibiotic therapy STAT[1]

Obtain CT scan of head. Is a mass lesion present?

No

Yes → Consider alternative diagnosis

Is cerebrospinal fluid consistent with Bacterial Meningitis?
- > 5 WBC, predominantly PMNs
- Glucose < 50 mg/dl or < 50% of serum
- Protein > 50 mg/dl
- Opening pressure > 20 cm H_2O

No → Consider alternative diagnosis

Yes → **Is the cerebrospinal fluid Gram stain or bacterial antigen test positive?**

Targeted Antimicrobial Therapy

Presumptive microorganism	Antimicrobial Therapy
Hemophilus influenzae type b	• Either cefotaxime 2g q4h or q6h or ceftriaxone 2 g q 12h.
Streptococcus pneumoniae	• Vancomycin 1 g q8h or q12h plus either cefotaxime or ceftriaxone .
Neisseria meningitidis	• Either Penicillin G 4 mU q4h or ampicillin 2 g q4h or cefotaxime or ceftriaxone
Listeria monocytogenes	• Ampicillin or penicillin G • If pen allergy, Trimethoprim-sulfamethoxazole 5 mg/kg q6 or q12h • Consider adding an aminoglycoside (gentamicin or tobramycin 1-1.5 mg/kg q8h or amikacin 5 mg/kg q8h)
Streptococcus agalactiae	• Ampicillin or penicillin G. Consider adding an aminoglycoside.

Doses above for patients with normal renal function. See *Dosing and Renal Failure Adjustments for Commonly Prescribed Drugs*

Tunkel AR, Scheld WM. Acute bacterial meningitis. Lancet 1995; 346: 1675-1680

Tunkel AR, Scheld WM. Acute meningitis. In: Principles and Practice of Infectious Diseases 5th ed. Philadelphia: Churchill-Livingstone. 1999: 959-997

Empiric Antimicrobial Therapy[1]

Age of Patient	Recommended Therapy
18-50 years	• Either cefotaxime 2 g q4h or q6h or ceftriaxone 2 g q12h. • Add Ampicillin 2 g q4h if Listeria monocytogenes is suspected
> 50 years	• Either cefotaxime or ceftriaxone • Add Ampicillin 2 g q4h

Vancomycin should be added to empiric regimens when highly penicillin- or cephalosporin- resistant strains of *Streptococcus pneumoniae* are suspected.

Recommended Antimicrobial Therapy Following Microorganism Identification and Susceptibility Testing

Microorganism	Antimicrobial Therapy	Duration
Hemophilus influenza type b		
β-lactamase negative	Ampicillin	7 days
β-lactamase positive	Cefotaxime or ceftriaxone	7 days
Streptococcus pneumoniae		
pcn MIC < 0.1 µg/ml	Penicillin G or ampicillin	10-14 days
pcn MIC 0.1 – 1.0 µg/ml	Cefotaxime or ceftriaxone	10-14 days
pcn MIC ≥ 2.0 µg/ml	Vancomycin + either cefotaxime or ceftriaxone; consider adding rifampin	10-14 days
Neisseria meningitidis		
pcn MIC < 0.1 µg/ml	Penicillin G or ampicillin	7 days
pcn MIC 0.1 – 1.0 µg/ml	Cefotaxime or ceftriaxone	7 days
Streptococcus agalctiae	Ampicillin or penicillin G; consider	
Listeria monocytogenes	adding an aminoglycoside	14-21days

14j: Brain Death*

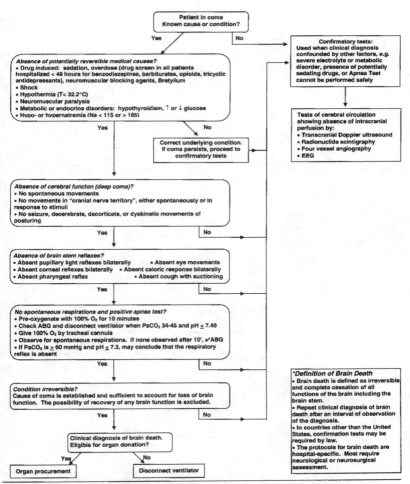

Patient in coma
Known cause or condition?

Yes → (continues down)
No → Confirmatory tests:

Confirmatory tests:
Used when clinical diagnosis confounded by other factors, e.g. severe electrolyte or metabolic disorder, presence of potentially sedating drugs, or Apnea Test cannot be performed safely

Tests of cerebral circulation showing absence of intracranial perfusion by:
- Transcranial Doppler ultrasound
- Radionuclide scintigraphy
- Four vessel angiography
- EEG

Absence of potentially reversible medical causes?
- Drug induced: sedation, overdose (drug screen in all patients hospitalized < 48 hours for benzodiazepines, barbiturates, opioids, tricyclic antidepressants), neuromuscular blocking agents, Bretylium
- Shock
- Hypothermia (T< 32.2°C)
- Neuromuscular paralysis
- Metabolic or endocrine disorders: hypothyroidism, ↑ or ↓ glucose
- Hypo- or hypernatremia (Na < 115 or > 165)

Yes → (continues down)
No → Correct underlying condition. If coma persists, proceed to confirmatory tests

Absence of cerebral functon (deep coma)?
- No spontaneous movements
- No movements in "cranial nerve territory", either spontaneously or in response to stimuli
- No seizure, decerebrate, decorticate, or dyskinetic movements of posturing

Yes / No

Absence of brain stem reflexes?
- Absent pupillary light reflexes bilaterally   • Absent eye movements
- Absent corneal reflexes bilaterally   • Absent caloric response bilaterally
- Absent pharyngeal reflex   • Absent cough with suctioning

Yes / No

No spontaneous respirations and positive apnea test?
- Pre-oxygenate with 100% O_2 for 10 minutes
- Check ABG and disconnect ventilator when $PaCO_2$ 34-45 and pH $\leq$ 7.40
- Give 100% O_2 by tracheal cannula
- Observe for spontaneous respirations. If none observed after 10', ✓ABG
- If $PaCO_2$ is $\geq$ 60 mmHg and pH $\leq$ 7.3, may conclude that the respiratory reflex is absent

Yes / No

Condition irreversible?
Cause of coma is established and sufficient to account for loss of brain function. The possibility of recovery of any brain function is excluded.

Yes / No

*Definition of Brain Death
- Brain death is defined as irreversible and complete cessation of all functions of the brain including the brain stem.
- Repeat clinical diagnosis of brain death after an interval of observation of the diagnosis.
- In countries other than the United States, confirmation tests may be required by law.
- The protocols for brain death are hospital-specific. Most require neurological or neurosurgical assessment.

Clinical diagnosis of brain death. Eligible for organ donation?

Yes → Organ procurement
No → Disconnect ventilator

Halevy A and Brody B. Brain death: Reconciling definitions, criteria, and tests. Ann Intern Med 119: 519-525, 1993
President's commission for the study of ethical problems in medicine and biomedical and behavioral research. Defining death: a report on the medical, legal, and ethical issues in the determination of death. Washington, DC. The Commission, 1981

14k: Depression

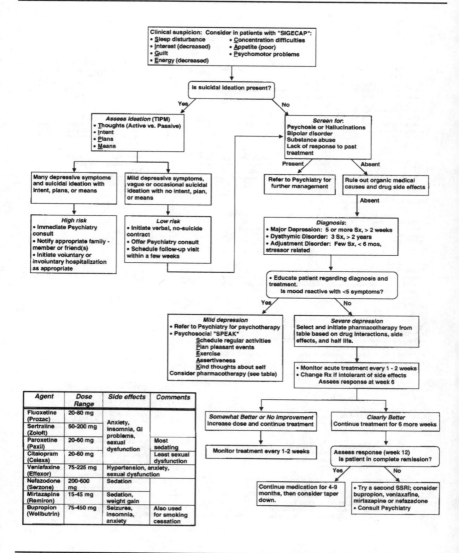

Clinical suspicion: Consider in patients with "SIGECAP":
- **S**leep disturbance
- **I**nterest (decreased)
- **G**uilt
- **E**nergy (decreased)
- **C**oncentration difficulties
- **A**ppetite (poor)
- **P**sychomotor problems

Is suicidal ideation present?

Yes → **Assess ideation (TIPM)**
- **T**houghts (Active vs. Passive)
- **I**ntent
- **P**lans
- **M**eans

No → **Screen for:**
Psychosis or Hallucinations
Bipolar disorder
Substance abuse
Lack of response to past treatment

Many depressive symptoms and suicidal ideation with intent, plans, or means

High risk
- Immediate Psychiatry consult
- Notify appropriate family - member or friend(s)
- Initiate voluntary or involuntary hospitalization as appropriate

Mild depressive symptoms, vague or occasional suicidal ideation with no intent, plan, or means

Low risk
- Initiate verbal, no-suicide contract
- Offer Psychiatry consult
- Schedule follow-up visit within a few weeks

Present → **Refer to Psychiatry for further management**

Absent → **Rule out organic medical causes and drug side effects**

Absent →

Diagnosis:
- Major Depression: 5 or more Sx, > 2 weeks
- Dysthymic Disorder: 3 Sx, > 2 years
- Adjustment Disorder: Few Sx, < 6 mos, stressor related

- Educate patient regarding diagnosis and treatment.
  Is mood reactive with <5 symptoms?

Yes → **Mild depression**
- Refer to Psychiatry for psychotherapy
- Psychosocial "SPEAK"
  - **S**chedule regular activities
  - **P**lan pleasant events
  - **E**xercise
  - **A**ssertiveness
  - **K**ind thoughts about self
Consider pharmacotherapy (see table)

No → **Severe depression**
Select and initiate pharmacotherapy from table based on drug interactions, side effects, and half life.

- Monitor acute treatment every 1 - 2 weeks
- Change Rx if intolerant of side effects
  Assess response at week 6

Somewhat Better or No improvement
Increase dose and continue treatment

Monitor treatment every 1-2 weeks

Clearly Better
Continue treatment for 6 more weeks

Assess response (week 12)
Is patient in complete remission?

Yes → Continue medication for 4-9 months, then consider taper down.

No →
- Try a second SSRI: consider bupropion, venlaxafine, mirtazapine or nefazodone
- Consult Psychiatry

Agent	Dose Range	Side effects	Comments
Fluoxetine (Prozac)	20-80 mg	Anxiety, insomnia, GI problems, sexual dysfunction	
Sertraline (Zoloft)	50-200 mg		
Paroxetine (Paxil)	20-60 mg		Most sedating
Citalopram (Celexa)	20-60 mg		Least sexual dysfunction
Venlafaxine (Effexor)	75-225 mg	Hypertension, anxiety, sexual dysfunction	
Nefazodone (Serzone)	200-600 mg	Sedation	
Mirtazapine (Remiron)	15-45 mg	Sedation, weight gain	
Bupropion (Wellbutrin)	75-450 mg	Seizures, insomnia, anxiety	Also used for smoking cessation

15a: Acne

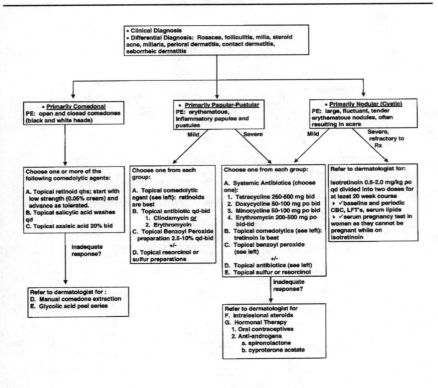

- Clinical Diagnosis
- Differential Diagnosis: Rosacea, folliculitis, milia, steroid acne, miliaria, perioral dermatitis, contact dermatitis, seborrheic dermatitis

• Primarily Comedonal
PE: open and closed comedones (black and white heads)

• Primarily Papular-Pustular
PE: erythematous, inflammatory papules and pustules

Mild / Severe

• Primarily Nodular (Cystic)
PE: large, fluctuant, tender erythematous nodules, often resulting in scars

Mild / Severe, refractory to Rx

Choose one or more of the following comedolytic agents:

A. Topical retinoid qhs; start with low strength (0.05% cream) and advance as tolerated.
B. Topical salicylic acid washes qd
C. Topical azaleic acid 20% bid

inadequate response?

Refer to dermatologist for :
D. Manual comedone extraction
E. Glycolic acid peel series

Choose one from each group:

A. Topical comedolytic agent (see left): retinoids are best
B. Topical antibiotic qd-bid
   1. Clindamycin or
   2. Erythromycin
C. Topical Benzoyl Peroxide preparation 2.5-10% qd-bid
   +/-
D. Topical resorcinol or sulfur preparations

Choose one from each group:

A. Systemic Antibiotics (choose one):
   1. Tetracycline 250-500 mg bid
   2. Doxycycline 50-100 mg po bid
   3. Minocycline 50-100 mg po bid
   4. Erythromycin 200-500 mg po bid-tid
B. Topical comedolytics (see left): tretinoin is best
C. Topical benzoyl peroxide (see left)
   +/-
D. Topical antibiotics (see left)
E. Topical sulfur or resorcinol

inadequate response?

Refer to dermatologist for
F. Intralesional steroids
G. Hormonal Therapy
   1. Oral contraceptives
   2. Anti-androgens
      a. spironolactone
      b. cyproterone acetate

Refer to dermatologist for:

Isotretinoin 0.5-2.0 mg/kg po qd divided into two doses for at least 20 week course
  ▸ ✓baseline and periodic CBC, LFT's, serum lipids
  ▸ ✓serum pregnancy test in women as they cannot be pregnant while on isotretinoin

Berger, TG et al. Manual of Therapy for Skin Diseases. New York: Churchill Livingstone, 1990.
Plewing, G and Kligman, AM. Acne and Rosacea. New York: Springer Verlag, 1993.
Leyden JJ. Therapy for acne vulgaris. N Engl J Med. 1997 Apr 17;336(16):1156-62. Review.
Brown SK, Shalita AR. Acne vulgaris. Lancet. 1998 Jun 20;351(9119):1871-6. Review.
Leyden JJ. Topical treatment of acne vulgaris: retinoids and cutaneous irritation. J Am Acad Dermatol. 1998, Apr;38(4): S1-4. Review.

15b: Fungal Infection of the Skin

A. Tinea Capitis	Choose one: a. Griseofulvin 250 mg po bid (microsized) or 125-187.5 mg po bid (ultramicrosized) for 4-6 weeks b. Itraconazole 100 mg po qd for 6 weeks c. Fluconazole 50 mg po qd for 10-20 days d. Terbenafine 250 mg po qd for 4-8 weeks

** treat affected family members and pets and dispose of contaminated combs, hats , etc.

B. Tinea Corporis and Cruris	1. Mild/localized cases: a. topical imidazole or allylamine products (econazole, miconazole, terbinafine, naftifine, etc.) 2. Severe/resistant cases (choose 1): a. Griseofulvin 125-187.5 mg ultramicrosized po bid (250mg microsized) for 2-4 weeks b. Nizoral 200 mg po qd for 3-6 weeks c. Itraconazole 100 mg po qd for 15 days d. Fluconazole 150 mg po qwk for 4 weeks e. Terbenafine 250 mg po qd for 2-4 weeks

**drying powders such as Zeabsorb and aeration may facilitate treatment

C. Tinea Manum D. Tinea Pedis	Same as T. Corporis but may require longer duration and higher doses

E. Tinea Unguium (Onychomycosis)	1. Topical therapies are usually not effective. Choose 1 oral agent below: a. Terbinafine 250 mg po qd for 6 weeks for fingernails, 12 weeks for toenails b. Itraconazole 200 mg po qd for 12 weeks, or 200mg po bid for one week of each month for 3-6 months c. Fluconazole 150 mg po qwk for up to 12 months d. Griseofulvin 250-375 mg ultramicrosized (500 mg po microsized) po bid for 4-9 months for fingernails, 6-18 months for toenails 2. Surgical or chemical nail plate avulsion followed by topical antifungal therapy

F. Tinea Versicolor	1. Mild/localized cases: a. Ketoconazole or selenium sulfide or zinc pyrithione or sulfur shampoos 2. Widespread/recalcitrant disease: a. Ketoconazole 200 mg po qd for one week or 400 mg po x1, repeat in one week b. Itraconazole 200 mg po qd for one week c. Fluconazole 400 mg po x1

G. Candidiasis (Intertrigo)	1. Mild/localized cases: a. Nystatin or imidazole preparations (topical econazoles, or systemic ketoconazole, etc.) b. Gentian violet or thymol preparations **keep area dry with powder (Zeabsorb) and aerated 2. Severe/recalcitrant cases: a. Ketoconazole 200 mg po qd for 1-2 weeks b. Itraconazole 100 mg po qd for 3-12 weeks c. Fluconazole 50 mg po qd

Dedoncker, P et al. Pulse therapy with one-week itraconazole monthly for three or four months in the treatment of onychomycosis. Cutis 1995;56:180-3.
Gupta, AK et al. Antifungal agents: An Overview. Part 1. J Am Acad Dermatol. 1994;30:677-98.
Gupta, AK et al. Antifungal agents: An Overview. Part 2. J Am Acad Dermatol. 1994;30:911-33.
Elewski BE. Update on superficial fungal infections. Introduction. Postgrad Med. 1999 Jul;Spec No:5.
Elewski BE. Tinea capitis: a current perspective. J Am Acad Dermatol. 2000 Jan;42(1 Pt 1):1-20.

15c: Psoriasis

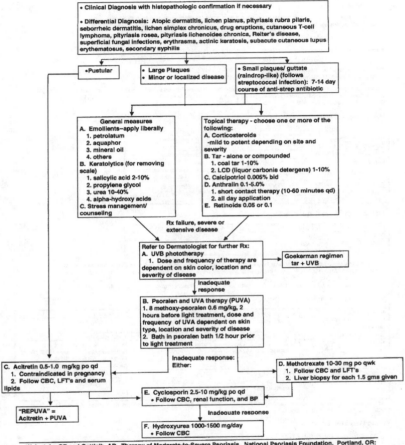

- Clinical Diagnosis with histopathologic confirmation if necessary
- Differential Diagnosis: Atopic dermatitis, lichen planus, pityriasis rubra pilaris, seborrheic dermatitis, lichen simplex chronicus, drug eruptions, cutaneous T-cell lymphoma, pityriasis rosea, pityriasis lichenoides chronica, Reiter's disease, superficial fungal infections, erythrasma, actinic keratosis, subacute cutaneous lupus erythematosus, secondary syphilis

- Pustular

- Large Plaques
- Minor or localized disease

- Small plaques/ guttate (raindrop-like) (follows streptococcal infection): 7-14 day course of anti-strep antibiotic

General measures
A. Emollients--apply liberally
1. petrolatum
2. aquaphor
3. mineral oil
4. others
B. Keratolytics (for removing scale)
1. salicylic acid 2-10%
2. propylene glycol
3. urea 10-40%
4. alpha-hydroxy acids
C. Stress management/ counseling

Topical therapy - choose one or more of the following:
A. Corticosteroids
 -mild to potent depending on site and severity
B. Tar - alone or compounded
1. coal tar 1-10%
2. LCD (liquor carbonis detergens) 1-10%
C. Calcipotriol 0.005% bid
D. Anthralin 0.1-5.0%
1. short contact therapy (10-60 minutes qd)
2. all day application
E. Retinoids 0.05 or 0.1

Rx failure, severe or extensive disease

Refer to Dermatologist for further Rx:
A. UVB phototherapy
1. Dose and frequency of therapy are dependent on skin color, location and severity of disease

Goekerman regimen tar + UVB

Inadequate response

B. Psoralen and UVA therapy (PUVA)
1. 8 methoxy-psoralen 0.6 mg/kg, 2 hours before light treatment, dose and frequency of UVA dependent on skin type, location and severity of disease
2. Bath in psoralen bath 1/2 hour prior to light treatment

Inadequate response: Either:

C. Acitretin 0.5-1.0 mg/kg po qd
1. Contraindicated in pregnancy
2. Follow CBC, LFT's and serum lipids

D. Methotrexate 10-30 mg po qwk
1. Follow CBC and LFT's
2. Liver biopsy for each 1.5 gms given

"REPUVA" = Acitretin + PUVA

E. Cyclosporin 2.5-10 mg/kg po qd
- Follow CBC, renal function, and BP

Inadequate response

F. Hydroxyurea 1000-1500 mg/day
- Follow CBC

Weinstein, GD and Gottlieb, AB. Therapy of Moderate-to-Severe Psoriasis. National Psoriasis Foundation. Portland, OR: Haber and Flora, Inc., 1993.
Greaves MW, Weinstein GD. Treatment of psoriasis. N Engl J Med 1995;332:581-8.
Linden KG, Weinstein GD. Psoriasis: current perspectives with an emphasis on treatment. Am J Med. 1999;107(6):595-605.
Lebwohl M. Advances in psoriasis therapy. Dermatol Clin. 2000 Jan;18(1):13-9, vii. Review.

16a: Nutrition Equations

Ideal body weight:

Females: 100 lb (45 kg) for first 5 ft (152 cm) plus 5 lb (2.3 kg) for each additional inch (2.54 cm)
Males: 106 lbs (48 kg) for first 5 ft (152 cm) plus 6 lbs (2.7 kg) for each additional inch

Caloric requirements:

Harris - Benedict equations:

Males: $REE = 66.47 + 13.75(IBW) + 5.0H - 6.76A$
Females: $REE = 655.1 + 9.5(IBW) + 9.56H - 4.88A$

Ireton-Jones equation for obese patients: $EE = 606S + 9W - 12A + 400V + 1,444$
Ireton-Jones equation for ventilator patients: $EE = 1925 - 10A + 5W + 281 S + 292T + 851B$

REE – resting energy expenditure in kcal/day; needs to be corrected for stress. EE – energy expenditure in kcal/day (no stress correction required). IBW – ideal body weight (kg); H – height in cm, A – age in years, S – sex (1=male, 0=female), T – trauma (0=absent, 1 = present), B – burn (0 = absent, 1 = present)

Weight based calculations:

Disease state	Estimate of caloric requirements
Usual maintenance diet	20-25 kcal/kg/day
Obesity (weight loss desired)	15-20 kcal/kg/day
Mild to moderate illness	25-35 kcal/kg/day
Renal disease	maintenance: 35 kcal/kg/day weight gain: 40-50 kcal/kg/day weight loss: 25-30 kcal/kg/day
Sepsis, multiorgan system failure, trauma	30-35 kcal/kg/day
Chylothorax, head trauma	35-45 kcal/kg/day
Pancreatitis, inflammatory bowel disease	45-50 kcal/kg/day

Methods of indirect calorimetry:

Weir equation for indirect calorimetry	$MEE = 1.44 (3.9\ VO_2 + 1.1\ VCO_2)$
Sherman equation using mixed expired CO2	$MEE = 9.27\ (PECO_2)(VE)$
Ligget - St. John - LeFrak equation using thermodilution cardiac output	$MEE = 95.18\ (CO)\ (Hb)\ (SaO_2\text{-}SvO_2)$

MEE = measured energy expenditure in kcal/day. VO_2 oxygen consumption in ml/min, VCO_2 – carbon dioxide production in ml/min. $PECO_2$ – partial pressure of expired carbon dioxide (collect several liters of expired gas in nonpermeable bag, mix, withdraw 10 cc and analyze with blood gas machine); VE – minute ventilation in liters/min. CO – cardiac output (l/m), Hb – hemoglobin; SaO_2 and SvO_2 are arterial and mixed venous saturations respectively.

Estimated Protein Requirements:

Minimal intake	0.54 g/kg/day	Cancer	1.5 g/kg/day
Recommended (RDA) intake	0.80 g/kg/day	COPD with malnutrition	1.5 - 2.0 g/kg/day
Catabolic States	1.2 - 1.6 g/kg/day	HIV infection	1 - 1.2 g/kg/day
Multiorgan system failure	Stable: 1.2 - 1.5 g/kg/day Stressed: 2.0 g/kg/day	Renal disease	No dialysis: 0.6 g/kg/day Hemodialysis: increase to1.2 g/kg/d Peritoneal dialysis: 1.2-1.5 CAVHD: 1.5-1.8
Trauma	1.5 - 2.0 g/kg/day	Chylothorax	1.5 - 2.0 g/kg/day
Hepatic cirrhosis	1.5 g/kg/day dry weight If encephalopathic: 0.5 - 0.7 g/kg/d dry weight	Pancreatitis/inflammatory bowel disease	1.3 - 2.0 g/kg/day

Adjust above to aim for Nitrogen Balance of +2-4 g/day: Nitrogen balance = 0.16 (g protein intake/day) - (UUN + 4)
UUN – 24 hour urine urea nitrogen.

Fluid Requirements:

1. 35 ml/kg body weight OR
2. 1500 ml/m^2 body surface area
3. Add 150 ml/day for every degree over 37°C

Aspen Board of Directors. Guideline for the use of parenteral nutrition in adult and pediatric patients. JPEN 17(4S):7-26SA, 1993
Gottschilich MM, Matarese LE, Shronts EP. Nutrition Support Core Curriculum, Aspen Publications, 1993
Schiltig et al., Nutritional Support of the critically ill. Yearbook Medical Publishers, Chicago, 1988

16b: Selecting an Enteral Formula

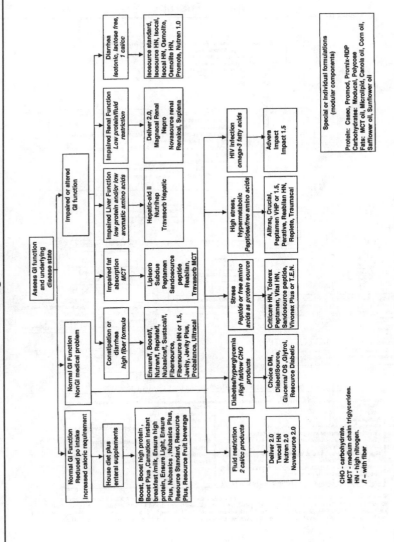

Assess GI function and underlying disease state

Normal GI Function

Normal GI Function
Reduced po intake
Increased caloric requirement
→ House diet plus enteral supplements
- Boost, Boost high protein, Boost Plus, Carnation instant breakfast/milk, Ensure high protein, Ensure Light, Ensure Plus, Nubasics, Nubasics Plus, Resource Standard, Resource Plus, Resource Fruit beverage

Normal GI Function NonGI medical problem

Constipation or diarrhea
high fiber formula
- Ensure/f, Boost/f, Nutren/f, Replete/f, Nubasics/f, Sustacal/f, Fibersource, Fibersource HN or 1.5, Jevity, Jevity Plus, Probalance, Ultracal

Fluid restriction
2 cal/cc products
- Deliver 2.0, Twocal HN, Nutren 2.0, Novasource 2.0

Diabetes/hyperglycemia
High fat/low CHO products
- Choice DM, DiabetiSource, Glucerna/OS, Glytrol, Resource Diabetic

Stress
Peptide or free amino acids as protein source
- Criticare HN, Tolerex, Peptamen, Vital HN, Sandosource peptide, Vivonex Plus or T.E.N.

High stress, Hypermetabolic
Peptides/free amino acids
- Alitra Q, Cruciat, Peptamen VHP or 1.5, Perative, Reabilan HN, Replete, Traumacal

HIV infection
omega-3 fatty acids
- Advera, Impact, Impact 1.5

Impaired or altered GI function

Impaired fat absorption
MCT
- Lipisorb, Subdue, Peptamen, Sandosource peptide, Reabilan, Travasorb MCT

Impaired Liver Function
low protein and/or low aromatic amino acids
- Hepatic-aid II, Nutrihep, Travasorb Hepatic

Impaired Renal Function
Low protein/fluid restriction
- Deliver 2.0, Magnacal Renal, Nepro, Novasource renal, Renalcal, Suplena

Diarrhea
Isotonic, lactose free, 1 cal/cc
- Isosource standard, Isosource HN, Isocal, Isocal HN, Osmolite, Osmolite HN, Promote, Nutren 1.0

Special or Individual formulations (modular components)

Protein: Casec, Promod, Promix-RDP
Carbohydrates: Moducal, Polycose
Fats: MCT oil, Microlipid, Canola oil, Corn oil, Safflower oil, Sunflower oil

CHO - carbohydrate.
MCT - medium chain triglycerides.
HN - high nitrogen.
/f - with fiber

Nutritional Assessment and Selection of Nutritional Support Therapy

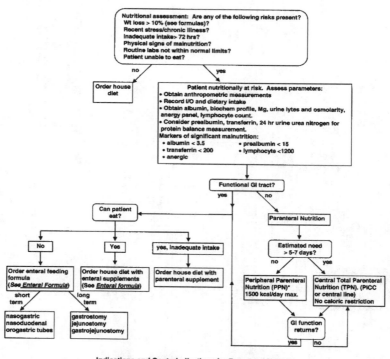

Nutritional assessment: Are any of the following risks present?
Wt loss > 10% (see formulas)?
Recent stress/chronic illness?
Inadequate intake> 72 hrs?
Physical signs of malnutrition?
Routine labs not within normal limits?
Patient unable to eat?

no → Order house diet

yes → Patient nutritionally at risk. Assess parameters:
• Obtain anthropometric measurements
• Record I/O and dietary intake
• Obtain albumin, biochem profile, Mg, urine lytes and osmolarity, anergy panel, lymphocyte count.
• Consider prealbumin, transferrin, 24 hr urine urea nitrogen for protein balance measurement.
Markers of significant malnutrition:
• albumin < 3.5   • prealbumin < 15
• transferrin < 200   • lymphocyte <1200
• anergic

Functional GI tract?

yes → Can patient eat?
- No → Order enteral feeding formula (See *Enteral Formula*)
  - short term → nasogastric, nasoduodenal, orogastric tubes
  - long term → gastrostomy, jejunostomy, gastrojejunostomy
- Yes → Order house diet with enteral supplements (See *Enteral formula*)
- yes, inadequate intake → Order house diet with parenteral supplement

no → Parenteral Nutrition
- Estimated need > 5-7 days?
  - no → Peripheral Parenteral Nutrition (PPN)* 1500 kcal/day max.
    - GI function returns? yes / no
  - yes → Central Total Parenteral Nutrition (TPN). (PICC or central line) No caloric restriction

Indications and Contraindications for Parenteral Nutrition

Indications	Contraindications
Bowel obstruction	Functioning GI tract
Ileus	Hemodynamically unstable
Hematemesis	No safe venous access
Chronic/intractable vomiting/diarrhea	Aggressive nutritional support not warranted by prognosis
Bowel rest (severe pancreatitis, chylous fistula)	Patient does not want aggressive nutritional support
High output or enterocutaneous fistulas	Treatment with TPN not anticipated for > 5-7 days in patients without malnutrition
Severe malabsorbtion	
Significant catabolism and prolonged NPO or clear fluid status (>5-7 days)	
Exacerbation of inflammatory bowel disease (short term)	
Short Bowel Syndrome (initially)	
Acute radiation, chemotherapy, or graft vs. host enteritis	

*PPN orders: 1 – 1.5 liters total volume (=1000 to 1500 kcal/d). Lipid: 500 – 800 kcal, CHO: 1000-1900 kcal, Protein: 45 g/L, N2: 7.15 g/L, Na: 36 meq/L, Cl: 35 meq/L, K 30 meq/L, Ca 4.7 meq/L, Mg 5 meq/L, Phos: 5-15 mMol/L, Acetate: 0-70 mEq/L. (or if your order entry requires salts instead of individual elements: NaCl 54 meq/L, KPhos 35 mmol/L, KCl 20 meq/L, MgSO4 10 meq/L. Ca gluconate 9.6 meq/L.: acetate can be given as Na- or K-acetate) to run at 40 ml/hr (1 liter) or 60 ml/hr (1.5 liters).

16d: Suggested TPN Orders

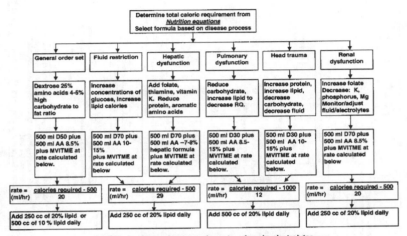

Determine total caloric requirement from *Nutrition equations*
Select formula based on disease process

General order set
Dextrose 25% amino acids 4-5% high carbohydrate to fat ratio
500 ml D50 plus 500 ml AA 8.5% plus MVITME at rate calculated below.
rate = $\dfrac{\text{calories required} - 500}{20}$ (ml/hr)
Add 250 cc of 20% lipid or 500 cc of 10% lipid daily

Fluid restriction
Increase concentrations of glucose, increase lipid calories
500 ml D70 plus 500 ml AA 10-15% plus MVITME at rate calculated below
rate = $\dfrac{\text{calories required} - 500}{29}$ (ml/hr)
Add 250 cc of 20% lipid daily

Hepatic dysfunction
Add folate, thiamine, vitamin K. Reduce protein, aromatic amino acids
500 ml D70 plus 500 ml AA −7-8% hepatic formula plus MVITME at rate calculated below.

Pulmonary dysfunction
Reduce carbohydrate, increase lipid to decrease RQ.
500 ml D30 plus 500 ml AA 8.5-15% plus MVITME at rate calculated below.
rate = $\dfrac{\text{calories required} - 1000}{12}$ (ml/hr)
Add 500 cc of 20% lipid daily

Head trauma
Increase protein, increase lipid, decrease carbohydrate, decrease fluid
500 ml D30 plus 500 ml AA 10-15% plus MVITME at rate calculated below.

Renal dysfunction
Increase folate Decrease: K, phosphorus, Mg Monitor/adjust fluid/electrolytes
500 ml D70 plus 500 ml AA 8.5% plus MVITME at rate calculated below
rate = $\dfrac{\text{calories required} - 500}{20}$ (ml/hr)
Add 250 cc of 20% lipid daily

MVITME -- multivitamins, trace elements, minerals, electrolytes

Vitamin	IV dose/day	Additive	IV dose	Trace elements	IV dose/day
Vit A	3300 IU	Cobalamin (B12)	5.0 µg/day	Chromium	10-15 mcg
Vit C	200 IU	Ascorbic acid (C)	100 mg/day	Copper	0.05-1.5 mg
Vit E	10 IU	Vit K*	2.5 mg/day	Iodine	1-2 mcg/kg
Thiamine (B1)	3.0 mg	Potassium[1]	60-100 mEq/l	Manganese	0.15-0.8 mg
Riboflavin (B2)	3.6 mg	Sodium[1]	60-130 mEq/l	Selenium	30-200 mcg
Niacin (B3)	15 - 40 mg	Acetate[2]	0–130 mEq/l	Zinc[3]	2.5-5.0 mg
Pantothenic acid (B5)	15 - 40 mg	Calcium[1]	5-15 mEq/l	Iron	1-2.5 mg
Pyridoxine (B6)	4.0 mg	Phosphorus[1]	15-45 mEq/l	Molybdenum	20 mcg
Biotin (B7)	60.0 mg	Magnesium[1]	10-30 mEq/l		
Floacin (B9)	400.0 µg	Chloride[1]	60-130 mEq/l		

*Vitamin K can be given as 10 mg weekly; do not give to patients on coumadin
1. check serum levels and adjust. Sodium is usually given as NaCl. Add (or replace NaCl with) Na acetate starting at 40 mEq/liter if serum CO2 < 25 meq/liter and adjust based on serum CO2 response. Do not exceed 150 mEq Na/L.
 • Add K as KCl if serum CO2>25mEq/l; add K as K acetate if serum CO2 < 25 mEq/l.
 • Calcium is usually given as Ca gluconate. Add 9 mEq/l if serum Ca < 8.5 meq/l; add 4.5 mEq/l if serum Ca > 8.5 meq/L; do not exceed 27 mEq/day.
2. Use for correction of acidosis in patients without hepatic dysfunction. May give as Na acetate or K acetate. K acetate should not exceed 40 meq/l.
3. Additional zinc may be required in acute catabolism (2mg/day), small bowel fluid losses (12.2 mg/liter fluid loss), and diarrhea/ileostomy output (17.1 mg/kg of output)

Nutritional values of intravenous sources

Solution	Kcal/Liter	Solution	kcal/cc	kcal/250 ml	crystalline amino acids	grams/liter
5% dextrose	170	10 % lipid	1.1	275	5.5%	55
10% dextrose	340	20% lipid	2.0	500	8.5%	85
30% dextrose	1020	30% lipid	3.0	750	10%	100
50% dextrose	1700				15%	150
70% dextrose	2380				8.0% hepatic	90

Grant J. Handbook of Total Parenteral Nutrition, 2nd ed. WB Saunders, Phila, PA, 1992.
Sheldon et. al., Electrolyte requirements in total parenteral nutrition. In: Nutrition in Clinical Surgery, Dietel M (ed), 1985
Schiltig et al. Nutritional Support of the Critically Ill. Yearbook Medical Publishers, Chicago 1988
Nutrition advisory group on standards and practice guidelines for parenteral nutrition special report: Safe practices for parenteral nutrition formulations. J Parenter Enter Nutr 22:2, 1998

17a: Initial Management of Oral Overdoses

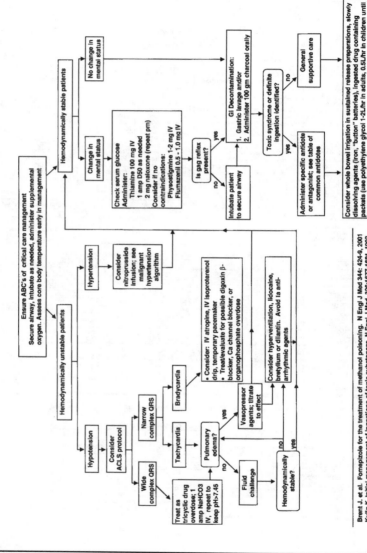

Brent J. et al. Fomepizole for the treatment of methanol poisoning. N Engl J Med 344: 424-9, 2001
Kulig K. Initial management of ingestions of toxic substances. N Engl J Med, 326;1677-1681, 1992.
Flomenbaum NE, et al. General management of the poisoned or overdosed patient. In Goldfrank LR et al (eds) Goldfrank's Toxicologic Emergencies, 5th ed., Appleton & Lange, Norwalk, 1994, p 25-42

17b: Common Antidotes

Acetaminophen	N-acetylcysteine: 140 mg/kg oral loading dose, 70 mg/kg po q4h x 17 doses
Anticholinergic agents	Physostigmine: 1-2 mg IV over 5 minutes, repeat as needed
Benzodiazepines	Flumazenil: 0.2-0.5 mg IV over 1minute Repeat until effect or up to 5 mg Note: Flumazenil may precipitate seizures in patients with chronic benzodiazepine or tricyclic antidepressant use.
Beta-blockers	Glucagon: 5-10 mg IV titrate to response Maintenance dose of 2-10 mg may be needed
Calcium channel blockers	Calcium chloride: 1 gm IV over 5 minutes May be repeated often in life-threatening cases Monitor calcium levels
Coumadin	Vitamin K1: 1.5-10mg IV (at 1mg/min), IM, SQ q4-8h, May repeat in 4-8 hrs per protimes.
Cyanide	Eli Lily Kit Amyl nitrite ampules broken and inhaled Sodium nitrite 10cc of 3% solution IV over 5 minutes Sodium thiosulfate 50cc of 25% solution IV over 10 minutes

Digitalis	Digibind: if unknown amount, begin with 10 vials
	If known amount, give as number of vials =
	   (mg of digoxin ingested divided by 0.6)
	If steady state serum level known, number of vials =
	   [concentration (ng/ml) x 5.6 x weight (kg)] divided by 600

Ethylene glycol	Ethanol: 10cc of 10% solution/kg IV loading dose, 0.15cc/kg/hr maintenance dose (see *Management of Suspected Toxic Alcohol Ingestion*)
Isoniazid	Pyridoxine: If unknown amount, give 5 mg IV + titrate upward If known, equivalent amounts i.e. give mg per mg ingested
Methanol	see ethylene glycol and *Management of Suspected Toxic Alcohol Ingestion*
Opiates	Naloxone: 0.4-2.0 mg IV initially Titrate upward until effect or until 10 mg is reached without effect
Organophosphates	Atropine: 2 mg IV, titrate upward to dry secretions, may require large doses Pralidoxime:25-50 mg/kg over 5 minutes, may require repeat dosing within 6 H
Tricyclic antidepressants	Sodium bicarbonate: 1-2 mmol/kg IV for cardiac dysrhythmia, repeat as needed. Consider physostigmine (above) for atrial arrhythmias/ conduction disturbances and CNS depression

Kulig K. Initial management of ingestions of toxic substances. N Engl J Med, 326(25);1677-1681, 1992.

17c: Management of Unknown Alcohol Ingestion

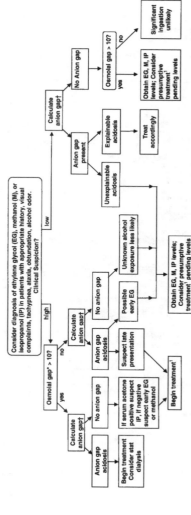

Consider diagnosis of ethylene glycol (EG), methanol (M), or isopropanol (IP) in patients with appropriate history, visual complaints, tachypnea, ataxia, obtundation, alcohol odor. Clinical Suspicion?

*Osmolal gap = serum measured osmolality – calculated osmolarity [2Na+(BUN/2.8)+(glucose/18) + (ethanol/4.6)] ≥ 10 mosm = abnormal.
Alcohols, acetone, beta-hydroxy-butyrate, acetoacetate, lactate, mannitol, hyperlipidemia, hyperprothrombinemia will all elevate osmolal gap
AG acidosis = anion gap acidosis
†Anion gap: Na – (Cl+HCO3). The upper limit of normal will vary with the laboratory, check with your laboratory normals. Usual value=12 ± 3.

1. Treatment = obtain stat EG, M, IP levels
   Administer fomepizole (Antizol) 15 mg/kg bolus, then 10 mg/kg q12h X 4 doses, each infusion over 30 minutes.
   If fomepizole not available, then begin ethanol therapy (assume 0 level at start, maintain serum level at 100-150 mg/dl):
   • If not fluid overloaded
     ‣ 10cc of 10% ethanol per kg, maintenance of 0.15 ml/ kg/hr
     ‣ In 70 kg person using 10% ethanol solution, load intravenously with 700 cc over 1-2 hours, maintain at 100 cc/hr
     ‣ Double volume if using 5 % ethanol solution
   • If fluid overloaded
     ‣ In 70 kg person using 80 proof, load with 175 cc orally, maintain at 30 cc/hr
   Administer thiamine, pyridoxine, folate
   Check ethanol and glucose levels frequently

Glaser DS. Utility of the serum osmol gap in the diagnosis of methanol or ethylene glycol ingestion. Ann Emerg Med. 1996 Mar;27(3):343-6.
Howland MA, Quattrocchi E. Commonly used infusion rates in Roberts JR, Hedges JR (eds) *Clinical Procedures in Emergency Medicine, 2nd ed.* WB Saunders, Philadelphia, 1991, p 1126-1127.

18a: Infusions Commonly Used in the ICU

DRUG	USUAL DOSE	STANDARD DILUTION [concentrated dilution]	STANDARD CONCENTRATION [concentrated]	SOLUTION	RATE (ml/hr) (ml/kg/hr)* [concentrated]*	MAXIMUM DOSE
Abciximab	Bolus: 0.25 mg/kg. Infuse: 0.125 µg/kg/min for up to 24 hours	Bolus: Varies / Drip: 9 mg/250 ml	Bolus: Varies / Drip: 0.036 mg/ml	D5W or NSS	0.208*	10 µg/min (17 ml/min)
Albumin	Expand plasma volume: 5% / Increase oncotic pressure: 25%	12.5 g/250 ml [25 g/100 ml]	0.05 g/ml [0.25 g/ml]	Undiluted; may use D5W or NSS	Rapidly, or 60 – 240 ml/hr (5%)	250 g/48 hrs
Amiodarone HCl	Bolus: 150mg over 10 min. Infuse: (1) 1 mg/min for 6 hr; then (2) 0.5 mg/min	Bolus: 150 mg/100ml / 900mg/500ml	Bolus: 1.5 mg/ml / Drip: 1.8 mg/ml	D5W only	Bolus: 600 (1) 33.3; (2)16.7	1 mg/min
Amrinone Lactate	Bolus: 0.75mg/kg over 2-3 min. Infuse: 5-20 mcg/kg/min	500mg/250ml	2 mg/ml	NSS only	Varies	18 mg/kg/day
Antithymocyte globulin–equine	Test dose: 0.1 ml of 1:1000 dilution, then 15 mg/kg/d (range 10-30) over at least 4 hours	Varies	Varies [max = 4 mg/ml]	NSS only	Varies	Varies
Antithymocyte globulin–rabbit	1.5 mg/kg/day (range 1-4) over at least 6 hours on day 1, then over at least 4 hours on remaining days	Varies	Varies ≤ 0.5 mg/ml	D5W or NSS	Varies	Varies
Bretylium	Bolus: 5 mg/kg then 10 mg/kg up to total of 30; Infuse: 1-2 mg/min	1000mg/250ml	4 mg/ml	D5W or NSS	15-30	40 mg/kg/day
Bumetanide	1-4 mg/hr	24mg/96ml	0.25 mg/ml	Undiluted	4-16	8 mg/hr
Cisatracurium Besylate	Bolus: 0.15-0.2 mg/kg. Infuse: 1-5 mcg/kg/min (0.06-0.3 mg/kg/hr)	400mg/200ml	2 mg/ml	D5W or NSS	0.03-0.15*	Titrate
Cyclosporin	1/3 usual oral dose over 24 hr	100ml	Varies	D5W	Varies	Varies
Diazepam	5-10 mg/hr	50mg/250ml [500mg/100ml]	0.2 mg/ml [5 mg/ml]	NSS [Undiluted]	25-50 [1-2]	Titrate
Diltiazem HCl	5-15 mg/hr	125mg/125ml	1 mg/ml	D5W or NSS	5-15	15 mg/hr
Dobutamine HCl	2.5-20 mcg/kg/min (0.15-1.2 mg/kg/hr)	500mg/250ml [1000mg/250ml]	2 mg/ml [4 mg/ml]	D5W or NSS	0.075-0.6* [0.0375-0.3]	40 mcg/kg/min
Dopamine HCl	1-20 mcg/kg/min (0.06-1.2 mg/kg/hr)	400mg/250ml [3200mg/250ml]	1.6 mg/ml [12.8 mg/ml]	D5W or NSS	0.0375-0.75* [0.0047-0.094]	40 mcg/kg/min
Epinephrine HCl	1-10 mcg/min	2 mg/250ml [16mg/250ml]	0.008mg/ml [0.064 mg/ml]	D5W or NSS	7.5-75 [0.94-9.4]	20 mcg/min
Eptifibatide	Non-ST segment elevation acute coronary syndrome (ACS) bolus: 180 µg/kg, then 2 µg/kg/min. Percutaneous coronary intervention (PCI) bolus: 135 µg/kg, then 0.5 µg/kg/min. Boluses over 1-2 minutes	Boluses: Vary / Infusions: 75 mg/100 ml	Boluses: 2 mg/ml / Infusions: 0.75 mg/ml	Premixed	ACS = 0.16* / PCI = 0.04*	22.6 mg bolus 15 ml/hr infusion (20 ml/hr)

18a: Infusions Commonly Used in the ICU (Cont.)

DRUG	USUAL DOSE	STANDARD DILUTION [concentrated dilution]	STANDARD CONCENTRATION [concentrated]	SOLUTION	RATE (ml/hr) (ml/kg/hr)* [concentrated]	MAXIMUM DOSE
Esmolol HCl	Bolus: 500 mcg/kg Infuse: 50-200 mcg/kg/min (3-12 mg/kg/hr)	5000mg/500ml [10,000mg/500ml]	10 mg/ml [20 mg/ml]	D5W or NSS	0.3-1.2* [0.15-0.6]	300 mcg/kg/min
Fenoldopam	0.01 – 1.5 µg/kg/min	1 mg/250 ml	0.04 mg/ml	D5W or NSS	0.015-2.25*	1.6µg/kg/min
Fentanyl Citrate	0.02-0.08 mcg/kg/min (0.0012-0.0048 mg/kg/hr)	2mg/250ml [4mg/250ml]	0.008 mg/ml [0.016 mg/ml]	D5W or NSS	0.15-0.6* [0.075-0.3]	Titrate
Furosemide	10-80 mg/hr	1000mg/100ml	10 mg/ml	Undiluted	1-8	240 mg/hr
Glucagon	1-5 mg/hr	Varies	Varies	D5W or NSS	Varies	5 mg/hr
Haloperidol Lactate	10 mg/hr	200mg/200ml [200mg/100ml]	1 mg/ml [2 mg/ml]	D5W	10 [5]	Titrate
Heparin Sodium	500-3200 Units/hr	25,000 Units/250ml	100 Units/ml	D5W or NSS	5-32	Titrate
Hetastarch	500-1000 ml per day	6% in 250 or 500 ml bags	60 mg/ml	Premixed	≤ 20 ml/kg/hr	1500 ml/day
Hydromorphone HCl	0.2-2 mg/hr	1 mg/ml [4 mg/ml]	1 mg/ml [4 mg/ml]	Undiluted	0.2-2 [0.05-0.5]	Titrate
Insulin Regular	0.1-0.2 Units/kg/hr	100 Units/100ml	1 Unit/ml	NSS	0.1-0.2*	Titrate
Isoproterenol HCl	Initiate: 5 mcg/min Range: 1-20 mcg/min	1mg/250ml [2mg/250ml]	0.004 mg/ml [0.008 mg/ml]	D5W or NSS	15-300 [7.5-150]	20 mcg/min
Labetalol HCl	Bolus: 20mg over 2 min then 40-80mg at 10 min intervals up to 300mg Infuse: 1-180 mg/hr	1000mg/200ml	5 mg/ml	D5W	0.2-36	Titrate
Lepirudin	Bolus: 0.4 mg/kg, then infuse 0.15 mg/kg/hr, adjust based on aPTT	Bolus: Varies 100 mg/500 ml [100 mg/250 ml]	Bolus: 5 mg/ml 0.2 mg/ml [0.4 mg/ml]	D5W or NSS	0.75* [0.375*]	44 mg bolus 16.5 mg/kg/hr infusion
Lidocaine HCl	Bolus: 1mg/kg Infuse: 1-4 mg/min	2000mg/250ml	8 mg/ml	D5W or NSS	7.5-30	4 mg/min
Lorazepam	1-8 mg/hr	1mg/ml	1 mg/ml	D5W only	1-8	12 mg/hr
Midazolam HCl	1-8 mg/hr	1mg/ml	1 mg/ml	Undiluted	1-8	20 mg/hr
Milrinone Lactate	Bolus: 50 mcg/kg over 10 min Infuse: 0.375-0.75 mcg/kg/min (0.0225-0.045 mg/kg/hr)	20mg/100ml [100mg/250ml]	0.2 mg/ml [0.4 mg/ml]	D5W or NSS	0.1125-0.225* [0.056-0.1125]	1.13 mg/kg/day
Morphine Sulfate	1-10 mg/hr	100mg/100ml	1 mg/ml	D5W or NSS	1-10	Titrate
Naloxone HCl	Overdose: Bolus 0.4 mg infuse: 0.25-6.25 mg/hr	2mg/500ml [10mg/100ml]	0.004 mg/ml [0.1 mg/ml]	D5W or NSS	62.5-1562.5 [2.5-62.5]	Titrate
Nicardipine HCl	Initiate: 5 mg/hr Range: 0.5-15 mg/hr	25mg/250ml	0.1 mg/ml	D5W or NSS	5-150	15 mg/hr
Nitroglycerin	5-250 mcg/min	50mg/250ml [150mg/250ml]	0.2 mg/ml [0.6 mg/ml]	D5W or NSS	1.5-75 [0.5-25]	Titrate

18a: Infusions Commonly Used in the ICU (Cont.)

DRUG	USUAL DOSE	STANDARD DILUTION [concentrated dilution]	STANDARD CONCENTRATION [concentrated]	SOLUTION	RATE (ml/hr)* [concentrated]	MAXIMUM DOSE
Norepinephrine Bitartrate	Initiate: 8-12 mcg/min Maintenance: 2-4 mcg/min	1mg/250ml [32mg/250ml]	0.004 mg/ml [0.128 mg/ml]	D5W or NSS	30-180 [0.94-1.88]	20 mcg/min
Octreotide Acetate	25-50 mcg/hr	500mcg/500ml [1000mcg/250ml]	1 mcg/ml [4 mcg/ml]	D5W or NSS	25-50 [6.25-12.5]	Titrate
Pancuronium Bromide	Bolus: 0.04-0.1 mg/kg over 1-2 min Infuse: 0.05 mg/kg/hr	20mg/250ml [40mg/250ml]	0.08mg/ml [0.16 mg/ml]	D5W or NSS	0.625* [0.3125]	Titrate
Pentobarbital Sodium	50 mg/min	2500mg/500ml	5 mg/ml	NSS	600	Titrate
Phenylephrine HCl	Initiate: 100-180 mcg/min Maintain: 40-60 mcg/min	10mg/500ml [60mg/250ml]	0.02 mg/ml [0.24 mg/ml]	D5W or NSS	120-540 [10-45]	Titrate
Phenytoin Sodium	Bolus: 15-20 mg/kg Infuse 25-50 mg/min	1000mg/250ml	4 mg/ml	NSS only	375-750	50 mg/min
Procainamide HCl	Bolus: 17 mg/kg over 1 hour Infuse Maintenance: 1-4 mg/min	2000mg/250ml [2000mg/100ml]	8 mg/ml [20 mg/ml]	D5W or NSS	7.5-30 [3-12]	6 mg/min (50 mg/kg/d)
Propofol	5-50 mcg/kg/min (0.3-3 mg/kg/hr)	1000mg/100ml	10 mg/ml	Premix	0.03-0.3*	Titrate
Prostaglandin E1	0.2-0.6 mcg/kg/hr	500mg/250ml	2 mcg/ml	D5W	0.1-0.3*	Titrate
Ranitidine HCl	6.25 mg/hr	150mg/150ml	1 mg/ml	D5W or NSS	6.25	400 mg/day
Sodium Nitroprusside	0.3-10 mcg/kg/min (0.018-0.6 mg/kg/hr)	50mg/250ml [150mg/250ml]	0.2 mg/ml [0.6 mg/ml]	D5W	0.09-3* [0.03-1]	10 mcg/kg/min
Tacrolimus	0.05-0.1 mg/kg/day over 24 hours	0.004-0.02mg/ml	Varies	D5W or NSS	Varies	Varies
Tirofiban	0.4 µg/kg/min for 30 minutes, then 0.1 µg/min for up to 108 hours	12.5 mg/250 ml	0.05 mg/ml	D5W or NSS	0.12-0.48*	Unknown
Trimethaphan Camsylate	0.3-6 mg/min	500mg/500ml	1 mg/ml	D5W or NSS	18-360	10 mg/min
Urokinase	Pulmonary embolism (PE): Bolus: 4,400 IU/kg Infuse: 4,400 IU/kg/hr for 12 hr Coronary Artery Thrombus (CAT): Bolus: 2,500-10,000 IU Infuse: 6,000 IU/min	PE: 2,000,000 IU/500ml CAT: 500,000 IU/250ml	PE: 4,000 IU/ml CAT: 2,000 IU/ml	D5W or NSS	PE: 1.1* CAT: 180	Varies
Vasopressin	0.1-0.4 Units/min	250 Units/250ml	1 Unit/ml	D5W	6-24	0.6 Units/min
Vecuronium Bromide	Bolus: 0.08-0.1 mg/kg Infuse: 0.05-0.1 mg/kg/hr	20mg/100ml [100mg/100ml]	0.2 mg/ml [1 mg/ml]	D5W or NSS	0.25-0.5* [0.05-0.1]	Titrate
Verapamil HCl	5-10 mg/hr	40mg/100ml	0.4 mg/ml	D5W or NSS	12.5-25	10 mg/hr

18b: #Rate Calculation (ml/hr) for Weight Based Dosing Regimens

Dose (ml/kg/hr)	Patient Weight					
	50 kg	60 kg	70 kg	80 kg	90 kg	100 kg
0.0047	0.235 ml/hr	0.282 ml/hr	0.329 ml/hr	0.376 ml/hr	0.423 ml/hr	0.47 ml/hr
0.015	0.75 ml/hr	0.9 ml/hr	1.05 ml/hr	1.2 ml/hr	1.35 ml/hr	1.5 ml/hr
0.03	1.5 ml/hr	1.8 ml/hr	2.1 ml/hr	2.4 ml/hr	2.7 ml/hr	3 ml/hr
0.0375	1.875 ml/hr	2.25 ml/hr	2.625 ml/hr	3 ml/hr	3.375 ml/hr	3.75 ml/hr
0.04	2 ml/hr	2.4 ml/hr	2.8 ml/hr	3.2 ml/hr	3.6 ml/hr	4 ml/hr
0.05	2.5 ml/hr	3 ml/hr	3.5 ml/hr	4 ml/hr	4.5 ml/hr	5 ml/hr
0.05625	2.8125 ml/hr	3.375 ml/hr	3.9375 ml/hr	4.5 ml/hr	5.0625 ml/hr	5.625 ml/hr
0.075	3.75 ml/hr	4.5 ml/hr	5.25 ml/hr	6 ml/hr	6.75 ml/hr	7.5 ml/hr
0.09	4.5 ml/hr	5.4 ml/hr	6.3 ml/hr	7.2 ml/hr	8.1 ml/hr	9 ml/hr
0.09375	4.69 ml/hr	5.6275 ml/hr	6.565 ml/hr	7.5 ml/hr	8.44 ml/hr	9.375 ml/hr
0.1	5 ml/hr	6 ml/hr	7 ml/hr	8 ml/hr	9 ml/hr	10 ml/hr
0.1125	5.625 ml/hr	6.75 ml/hr	7.875 ml/hr	9 ml/hr	10.125 ml/hr	11.25 ml/hr
0.12	6 ml/hr	7.2 ml/hr	8.4 ml/hr	9.6 ml/hr	10.8 ml/hr	12 ml/hr
0.15	7.5 ml/hr	9 ml/hr	10.5 ml/hr	12 ml/hr	13.5 ml/hr	15 ml/hr
0.16	8 ml/hr	9.6 ml/hr	11.2 ml/hr	12.8 ml/hr	14.4 ml/hr	16 ml/hr
0.2	10 ml/hr	12 ml/hr	14 ml/hr	16 ml/hr	18 ml/hr	20 ml/hr
0.225	11.25 ml/hr	13.5 ml/hr	15.75 ml/hr	18 ml/hr	20.25 ml/hr	22.5 ml/hr
0.25	12.5 ml/hr	15 ml/hr	17.5 ml/hr	20 ml/hr	22.5 ml/hr	25 ml/hr
0.3	15 ml/hr	18 ml/hr	21 ml/hr	24 ml/hr	27 ml/hr	30 ml/hr
0.3125	15.625 ml/hr	18.75 ml/hr	21.875 ml/hr	25 ml/hr	28.125 ml/hr	31.25 ml/hr
0.375	18.75 ml/hr	22.5 ml/hr	26.25 ml/hr	30 ml/hr	33.75 ml/hr	37.5 ml/hr
0.48	24 ml/hr	28.8 ml/hr	33.6 ml/hr	38.4 ml/hr	43.2 ml/hr	48 ml/hr
0.5	25 ml/hr	30 ml/hr	35 ml/hr	40 ml/hr	45 ml/hr	50 ml/hr
0.6	30 ml/hr	36 ml/hr	42 ml/hr	48 ml/hr	54 ml/hr	60 ml/hr
0.625	31.25 ml/hr	37.5 ml/hr	43.75 ml/hr	50 ml/hr	56.25 ml/hr	62.5 ml/hr
0.75	37.5 ml/hr	45 ml/hr	52.5 ml/hr	60 ml/hr	67.5 ml/hr	75 ml/hr
1	50 ml/hr	60 ml/hr	70 ml/hr	80 ml/hr	90 ml/hr	100 ml/hr
1.1	55 ml/hr	66 ml/hr	77 ml/hr	88 ml/hr	99 ml/hr	110 ml/hr
1.2	60 ml/hr	72 ml/hr	84 ml/hr	96 ml/hr	108 ml/hr	120 ml/hr
2.25	112.5 ml/hr	135 ml/hr	157.5 ml/hr	180 ml/hr	202.5 ml/hr	225 ml/hr
3	150 ml/hr	180 ml/hr	210 ml/hr	240 ml/hr	270 ml/hr	300 ml/hr

Anderson PO, Knoben JE. Handbook of Clinical Drug Data, 8th ed. Appleton & Lange, Stamford, 1997
McEvoy GK. AHFS Drug Information. American Society of Health-System Pharmacists, Bethesda, 1996
Trissel LA. Handbook on Injectable Drugs, 9th ed. American Society of Health-System Pharmacists, Bethesda,1996

18c: Therapeutic Drug Monitoring Guidelines for Selected Agents

Drug	Half-life (h)	Therapeutic Range	Potentially Toxic Range	Time to Steady-state[1]	When to Sample[2]
Aminoglycosides	Normal: 2-3h; Anephric: 30-60h	Gentamicin, Tobramycin, and Netilmicin[3]: peak 4-8 mg/L; trough<2 mg/L. Amikacin[3]: peak 20-30 mg/L; trough<10 mg/L	Gentamicin, Tobramycin, Netilmicin[3]: peak>10 mg/L; trough>2 mg/L. Amikacin[3]: peak>30 mg/L; trough>10 mg/L.	Normal: 12-24 h; Anephric: 6-12 d	Obtain peak and trough levels
Carbamazepine	15-20 h	4-12 mg/L	>12 mg/L	60-80 h	Trough
Chloramphenicol	4 h	Peak 15-25 mg/L; Trough 5-10 mg/L	Peak > 25 mg/L; Trough > 10 mg/L	18 h	Obtain peak 1 hour after the end of infusion
Cyclosporine	16-26h	100-400 μg/L	>400 μg/L	80-130h	IV: after 4 days of continuous IV therapy PO: trough level
Digoxin	24-36 h	CHF: 0.6-1.2 μg/L (0.7-1.4μmol/L); SVT: 0.9-2.0 μg/L (0.7-2.4μmol/L)	> 2.0 μg/L (>2.4μmol/L)	5-7 d	At least 12 h after dose given
Ethosuximide	30-50 h	40-100 mg/L	> 100 mg/L	180-250 h	Trough
5-flucytosine	4 h	35-70 mg/L	> 100 mg/L	20 h	Trough
Lidocaine	Normal: 1h; CHF: 4-6 h; CLD[4]: 6h	2-6 mg/L (6-21.5 μmol/L)	> 6 mg/L (> 21.5μmol/L)	6-24 h	At least 6h after start of infusion
Lithium	20 h	0.6-1.2 mEq/L	>1.5 mEq/L	100 h	Morning trough
Phenobarbital	5 d	10-30 mg/L	> 35 mg/L	20-30 d	Obtain trough at least 2-3 weeks after initiation of therapy or change in dose[5]
Phenytoin	75-125 h	10-20 mg/L (40-80 μmol/L)	>25 mg/L (>100 μmol/L)	7-14 d	Obtain trough at least 5-7 days after initiation or change in dose[5]
Phenytoin, free	75-125 h	1-2 mg/L (4-8 μmol/L)	>2.5 mg/L (>10 μmol/L)	7-14 d	Obtain only in patients with altered protein binding, e.g., renal failure, hepatic failure, malnutrition
Primidone	7 h	8-12 mg/L	>12 mg/L	35 h	Obtain trough level for primidone; also obtain trough level for phenobarbital (metabolite) 2-3 weeks after initiation of therapy or change in dose
Procainamide	P[6]: 3 h; NAPA: 6h	4-10 mg/L (P[6] only) (17-42.5 μmol/L)	>10 mg/L (P[6] only >42.5 μmol/L); >30 mg/L (P[6]+NAPA >127.5 μmol/L)	P[6]: 15 h; NAPA: 30h	IV: Sample 12h after initiation PO: Trough
Quinidine	6.5 h	2-5 mg/L (4.6-11.5 μmol/L)	>10 mg/L (>23 μmol/L)	30 h	Trough
Tacrolimus	15 h	5-8 ng/mL	>10 ng/mL	75 h	Trough
Theophylline	8.3 h	5-15 mg/L (27.5-85 μmol/L)	>20 mg/L	38-48 h	IV: anytime during the infusion PO: trough level
Valproic acid	6-12 h	50-100 mg/L	>100 mg/L	35-60 h	Trough
Vancomycin	Normal: 7 h; Anephric: 7 days	Peak: 30-50 mg/L; Trough: 5-15 mg/L	Peak: >50 mg/L; Trough: >20 mg/L	Normal: 30 h; Anephric: 14-28 d	Obtain peak and trough levels

Steady-state assumes stable physiologic status; [a]Obtain trough level just before the next dose. Obtain peak level one hour after end of infusion. [b]Higher peak levels may be necessary for more serious infections; [c]Chronic liver disease; [d]Procainamide, [e]Procainamide, Trough levels may be obtained more frequently in patients with acute illness (e.g. status epilepticus) in whom therapeutic levels need to be established quickly.

1. Evans WE, Schentag JJ, Jusko WJ, eds. Applied Pharmacokinetics, 3rd ed. Vancouver, WA: Applied Therapeutics, Inc., 1992.
2. Winter ME, ed. Basic Clinical Pharmacokinetics, 2nd ed. Vancouver, WA: Applied Therapeutics, Inc., 1988

18d: Dosing and Renal Failure Adjustments for Commonly Prescribed Drugs

Dosing and renal adjustments are listed below. Choose doses within an antibiotic range based on severity. For antihypertensives and oral diabetic agents, start at the low end of the range. Check references for additional information and other agents. Dose ranges are guidelines; dosages may require adjustment by drug level and clinical effect.
• GFR can be estimated using the Cockcroft/Gault formula: [(140-age) X ideal body weight in kg]/(72 X serum creatinine in mg/dl). Multiply by 0.85 for females. Formula can only be used if creatinine is stable. Assume oliguric patients to have a creatinine clearance < 10.
• Ideal body weight for men = 50 kg for first 5 feet, plus 2.3 kg for each additional inch.   • Ideal body weight for women = 45.5 kg for first 5 feet, plus 2.3 kg for each additional inch.

Antibiotics

1. Aminoglycosides

Drug	Normal	GFR > 50	GFR 10-50	GFR <10	Hemodialysis supplement
Amikacin/ Kanamycin	5 mg/kg q8h	3 - 4.5 mg/kg q12h	1.5 - 3.5 mg/kg q12 - 18 h	1 - 1.5 mg/kg q24 - 48 h	3.5 mg/kg post dialysis
Gentamicin/ Tobramycin	1-1.5 mg/kg q8h or 5 mg/kg/d	0.5 - 1 mg/kg q8-12h	0.3 - 0.7 mg/kg q12h	0.2-0.3 mg/kg q24-48h	0.7 mg/kg post dialysis
Streptomycin	1g qd	1 g qd	1g q24-72h	1g q72-96h	0.5 g post dialysis

2. Cephalosporins

Drug	Normal	GFR > 50	GFR 10-50	GFR<10	Hemodialysis supplement
Cefaclor	250 - 500 mg q8h or 375 - 500 mg extended release q12h	250 - 500 mg q8h or 375 - 500 mg extended release q12h	250 500 mg q8h or 375 - 500 mg extended release q12h	250 mg q8h or 375 mg extended release q12h	250 mg post dialysis
Cefadroxil	500 - 1000 mg q12h	500 - 1000 mg q12h	500 - 1000 mg q12 - 24h	500 - 1000 mg q24 - 48h	500 - 1000 mg post dialysis
Cefamandole	500 - 1000 mg q4 - 8h	500 - 1000 mg q6h	500 - 1000 mg q6 - 8h	500 - 1000 mg q12h	500 - 1000 mg post dialysis
Cefazolin	500 - 1500 mg q6h	500 - 1500 mg q6h	500 - 1500 mg q12h	500 - 1500 mg q24 - 48h	500 - 1000 mg post dialysis
Cefepime	250 - 2000 mg q8h	250 - 2000 mg q12h	250 - 2000 mg q12 - 16h	250 - 2000 mg q24 - 48h	1000 mg post dialysis
Cefixime	200 mg q12h or 400 mg qd	200 mg q12h or 400 mg qd	300 mg qd	200 mg qd	300 mg post dialysis
Cefonicid	1 g qd	500 mg qd	100 - 500 mg qd	100 mg qd	none
Cefotaxime	1 - 2 g q4 - 6h	1 - 2 g q6h	1 - 2 g q6-12h (PDR suggests half normal dose if GFR<20)	1 - 2 g q24h (PDR suggests half normal dose if GFR<20)	1 gram after dialysis
Cefotetan	1 - 2 g q12h	1 - 2 g q12h	1 - 2 g q24h (GFR < 30)	1 - 2 g q48h	1 gram after dialysis
Cefoxitin	1 - 2 g q6-8h	1 - 2 g q8h	1 - 2 g q8-12h	1 - 2 g q24-48h	1 gram after dialysis
Cefpodoxime	200 mg q12h	200 mg q12h	200 mg q16h	200 mg q24 - 48h	200 mg after dialysis
Ceftazidime	1 - 2 g q8h	1 - 2 g q8 - 12h	1 - 2 g q24 - 48h	1 - 2 g q48h	1 gram after dialysis
Ceftizoxime	1 - 2 g q8 - 12h	1 - 2 g q8 - 12h	1 - 2 g q24 - 48h	1 - 2 g q12 - 24h	1 gram after dialysis
Cefuroxime sodium	750 - 1500 mg q8h	750 -1500 mg q8h	750 mg q12h (GFR <20)	750 mg qd	Dose after dialysis
Cephalexin/ Cephradine	250 - 500 mg q6h	250 - 500 mg q6h	250 - 500 mg q12h	250 - 500 mg q24h	Dose after dialysis

No renal adjustment necessary: Cefoperazone (1- 2g q12h), Ceftriaxone (1 - 2 g qd; or 2 g q12h for meningitis), Cefuroxime axetil (250 - 500 mg q12h)

3. Macrolides/azalides

Drug	Normal	GFR > 50	GFR 10-50	GFR<10	Hemodialysis supplement
Clarithromycin	500 - 1000 mg q12h	500 -1000 mg q12h	500 - 750 mg q12h	250 - 750 mg q12h	Dose after hemodialysis
Erythromycin	250 - 500 mg q6-12h	250 -1000 mg q6-12h	250 - 1000 mg q6-12h	250 - 750 mg q6-12h	None

No renal adjustment necessary: Azithromycin (500 mg day 1, then 250 - 500 mg qd)

4. Penicillins

Drug	Normal	GFR > 50	GFR 10-50	GFR<10	Hemodialysis dose
Amoxicillin	250-500 mg q8h	250 - 500 mg q8h	250 - 600 mg q8-12h	250 - 500 mg qd	250 - 500 mg post dialysis
Ampicillin	250 mg - 2 g q6h	250 mg - 2 g q6h	250 mg - 2 g q6 - 12h	250 mg - 2 g q12-24h	250 mg - 2 g post dialysis
Amoxicillin/clavulanic acid	250 mg q8h or 500 - 875 mg q12h	250 mg q8h or 500 - 875 mg q12h	250 - 500 mg q12h	250 - 500 mg qd	250 - 500 mg during and post dialysis

18d: Dosing and Renal Failure Adjustments for Commonly Prescribed Drugs (Cont.)

Drug	Normal	GFR > 50	GFR 10-50	GFR<10	Hemodialysis dose
Ampicillin/sulbactam	1.5 - 3 g q6h	1.5 - 3 g q6 - 8h	1.5 - 3 g q8 - 12h	1.5 - 3 g qd	1.5 3 g post dialysis
Methicillin	1 - 2 g q4h	1 - 2 g q4 - 6h	1 - 2 g q6 - 8h	1 - 2 g q8 - 12h	none
Mezlocillin	1.5 - 4.0 g q 4 - 6h	1.5 - 4.0 g q 4 - 6h	1.5 - 4.0 g q 6 - 8h	1.5 - 4.0 g q 8 -12h	none
Penicillin G	0.5 - 4 milllion U q6h	0.5 - 4 milllion U q6h	0.375 - 3 million U q6h	0.2 - 2 million U q6h	0.5 - 4 million U post dialysis
Piperacillin	3 - 4 g q4h	3 - 4 g q4 - 6h	3 - 4 g q6 - 8h	3 - 4 g q8h	3 - 4 g post dialysis
Piperacillin/tazobactam	3.375 g q4-6h	3.375 g q6h	2.25 g q6h (GFR 20-50)	2.25 g 8 (GFR < 20)	2.25 q6, + 0.75 g post dialysis
Ticarcillin	3 g q4h		1 - 2g q8h	1 - 2g q12h	3g post dialysis
Ticarcillin/ clavulanic acid	3.1 g q4 - 6h	3.1 g q4 - 6h	2g q4 h (GFR 30 -60) 2 g q8h (GFR 10 - 30)	2g q12h	3.1 g post dialysis

No renal adjustment necessary: Nafcillin (1-2g q4-6h), Penicillin VK (250 - 500 mg q6h)

5. Quinolones

Drug	Normal	GFR > 50	GFR 10-50	GFR<10	Hemodialysis dose
Ciprofloxacin	500 - 750 mg q 12h po OR 200 – 400 mg q 12h IV	500 - 750 mg q 12h po OR 200 – 400 mg q 12h IV	250- 500 mg q 12h po OR 200 – 400 mg q 18 - 24h IV (GFR < 30)	250 - 375 mg q 12h po OR 200 – 400 mg q 18 - 24h IV	250 mg q12h po
Gatifloxacin	400 mg qd IV or po	400 mg qd	GFR < 40, 400 mg load, then 200 mg qd. No adjustment for 1 day Rx (gonorrhea) or 3 day Rx (uncomplicated UTI)		
Levofloxacin	250 - 500 mg qd (IV or po)	250 - 500 mg qd (IV or po)	500 mg load, then 250 mg qd (IV or po, GFR 20 - 50)	500 mg load, then 250 mg q48h (IV or po , GFR < 20)	Dose per GFR < 10, no supplement needed
Norfloxacin	400 mg po q12h	400 mg po q12h	400 mg po q12 - 24h	Avoid	Avoid
Ofloxacin	400 mg q 12	200 – 400 mg q12h	200 – 400 mg qd (GFR 20-50)	200-400 mg load then 100-200 mg qd (GFR < 20)	

No renal adjustment necessary: Moxifloxacin (500 mg qd)

6. Tetracyclines

Drug	Normal	GFR > 50	GFR 10-50	GFR<10	Hemodialysis dose
Tetracycline	250 - 500 mg qid	250 - 500 mg q8-12h	250 - 500 mg q12 - 24h	250 - 500 mg qd	no supplement

No renal adjustment necessary: Minocycline (100 mg q12h), Doxycycline (100 mg qd)

7. Miscellaneous antibacterials

Drug	Normal	GFR > 50	GFR 10-50	GFR-10	Hemodialysis dose
Aztreonam	1 - 2 g q6-12h	1 - 2 g q6-12h (GFR > 30)	1 - 2 g load, then 0.5 - 1 g q 8 -12h (GFR 10 - 30)	1 - 2 g load, then 250 - 500 mg q6-12h	0.5g post dialysis
Imipenem	250 - 1000 mg q6h	250 - 1000 mg q6h	250 - 500 mg q6h	250 mg q6h	Dose post dialysis
Meropenem	0.5 – 2.0 g q8h	0.5-2.0 g q 8h	1 g q 12h (GFR 25-50) 0.5 g q 12h (GFR 10-25)	0.5 g q 24h	0.5 g post dialysis
Metronidazole	7.5 mg/kg q6h	7.5 mg/kg q6h	7.5 mg/kg q6h	3.75 mg/kg q6h	Dose post dialysis
Nitrofurantoin	50 - 100 mg q6h	50 - 100 mg q6h	Avoid	Avoid	Avoid
Trimethoprim/sulfaxazole (severe UTI or Shigella)	8-10 mg/kg/day (TMP based) divided in q6 to q12h doses	8-10 mg/kg/day (TMP based) divided in q 6 to q12h doses	4-5 mg/kg/day (TMP) divided in q6 to q12h doses (GFR < 30)	Avoid	Avoid
Trimethoprim/sulfaxazole (Pneumocystis carinii)	15-20 mg/kg/day (TMP) divided in q6 or q6h doses	15 - 20 mg/kg/day (TMP) divided in q8 or q6h doses	7.5-10 mg/kg/day (TMP) divided in q8 or q6h doses (GFR< 30)	Avoid	Avoid
Vancomycin	500 mg q6h or 1g q12h	500 mg q6-12h	500mg q24-48h	500 mg q48-96h or 1 g q74, adjust dose for drug levels	500 mg q48-96h or 1 g q74, adjust dose for drug levels

No renal adjustment necessary: Chloramphenicol (12.5 mg/kg q6h), Clindamycin (150 - 300 mg q8h), Quinupristin/Dalfopristin (7.5 mg/kg q8-12h), Linezolid 400-600 mg q12h

149

18d: Dosing and Renal Failure Adjustments for Commonly Prescribed Drugs (Cont.)

8. Antifungals

Drug	Normal	GFR > 50	GFR 10-50	GFR <10	Hemodialysis dose
Amphotericin B	20 – 40 mg (or 0.25-1.5 mg/kg) qd	20 – 40 mg (or 0.25-1.5 mg/kg)qd	20 – 40 mg (or 0.25-1.5 mg/kg) qd	20 – 40 mg (or 0.25-1.5 mg/kg) q24-36h	none
Amphotericin B lipid complex	Abelcet 5 mg/kg qd Amphotec 3 - 4 mg/kg qd	No dose adjustment. Dosage interval may be extended depending on clinical condition of the patient.			
Flucytosine	37.5 mg/kg q6h	37.5 mg/kg q12h	37.5 mg/kg q16h	37.5 mg/kg qd	Dose after dialysis
Itraconazole	100 - 200 mg q12h	100 - 200 mg q12h	100 - 200 mg q12h	50 - 100 mg q12h	none

No renal adjustment necessary: Fluconazole (200 -400 mg qd; 200 mg after dialysis), Ketoconazole (200 mg qd), Miconazole (200 - 1200 mg q8h),

Antiviral agents

Drug	Normal	GFR > 50	GFR 10-50	GFR <10	Hemodialysis dose
Acyclovir	5 mg/kg q8h	5 mg/kg q8h	5 mg/kg q12-24h	2.5 mg/kg q24h	2.5 mg/kg post HD
Didanosine	≥ 60 mg: 200 mg q12h < 60 mg: 125 mg q12h	Recommendations not available	Recommendations not available	Recommendations not available	Recommendations not available
Ganciclovir (Induction IV)	5 mg/kg q12h	2.5 mg/kg q12h	2.5 mg/kg q24h (GFR 25-49) 1.25 mg/kg q24h (GFR 10-24)	1.25 mg/kg TIW	1.25 mg/kg TIW post dialysis
(Maintenance IV)	6 mg/kg q24h	2.5 mg/kg q24h	1.25 mg/kg q24h (GFR 25-49) 0.625 mg/kg q24h (GFR 10-24)	0.625 mg/kg TIW	0.625 mg/kg TIW post dialysis
(PO)	1000 mg q8h	500 mg q8h	500mg q12h (GFR 25-49) 500 mg q24h (GFR 10-24)	500 mg TIW	500 mg TIW post dialysis
Lamivudine	150 mg q12h	150 mg q12h	150 mg x1, then 100 mg qd (GFR 30-49) 150 mg x1, then 100 mg qd (GFR 15-29)	150 mg x1, then 50 mg qd (GFR 5-14) 50 mg x1 then 25 mg qd (GFR <5)	No recommendations
Nevirapine	200 mg q12h	Recommendations not available	Recommendations not available	Recommendations not available	Recommendations not available
Stavudine	≥ 60 kg: 40 mg q12h < 60 kg: 30 mg q12h	≥ 60 kg: 40 mg q12h < 60 kg: 30 mg q12h	≥ 60 kg: 20 mg q12h (GFR 26-50) < 60 kg: 15 mg q12h (GFR 26-50) ≥ 60 kg: 20 mg q24h (GFR 10-25) < 60 kg: 15 mg q24h (GFR 10-25)	Recommendations not available	Recommendations not available
Zalcitabine	0.75 mg q8h	0.75 mg q8h (GFR >40)	0.75 mg q12h (GFR 10-40)	0.75 mg q24h	Recommendations N/A
Zidovudine	200 mg q8h	200 mg q8h	200 mg q8h	100 mg q6-8	100 mg q6-8

No renal adjustment necessary: Indinavir (800 mg q8h), Nelfinavir (750 mg q8h), Ritonavir (600 mg q12h), Saquinavir (Invirase 600 mg q8h po; Fortovase 1200mg q8h po); Abacavir (300 mg q12h), Amprenavir (1200 mg q12h), Delavirdine (400 mg q8h), Efavirenz (600 mg qd)

Antihypertensive and Cardiovascular drugs
1. Adrenergic/serotonergic mediators

Drug	Normal	GFR > 50	GFR 10-50	GFR <10	Hemodialysis dose
Guanadrel	10 - 50 mg q12h	10 - 50 mg q12h	10 - 50 mg q12-24h	10 - 50 mg q24- 48h	unknown
Guanethidine	10 - 100 mg qd	10 - 100 mg qd	10 - 100 mg qd	10 - 100 mg q 24 - 48hh	unknown
Methyldopa	250 - 500 mg q 8h	250 - 500 mg q 8h	250 - 500 mg q 8 - 12h	250 - 500 mg q 12 - 24h	250 mg post dialysis
Reserpine	0.05 - 0.25 mg qd	0.05 - 0.25 mg qd	0.05 - 0.25 mg qd	avoid	avoid

No renal adjustment necessary: Clonidine (0.1 to 0.6 mg q12h, or TTS 1, 2, or 3 patch q week), Doxazosin (1 - 16 mg qd), Guanabenz (8 - 16 mg q12h), Ketanserin (40 mg q12h), Prazosin (1 - 15 mg q12h), Terazosin (1 - 20 mg qd)

2. Angiotensin converting enzyme inhibitors

Drug	Normal	GFR > 50	GFR 10-50	GFR<10	Hemodialysis dose
Benazepril	10 - 40 mg qd	10 - 40 mg qd	5 - 40 mg qd	5 - 20 mg qd	5 mg
Captopril	25 - 50 mg q8 - 12h	25 - 50 mg q8 - 12h	12.5 - 25 mg q12 - 18h	12.5 mg qd	6.25 mg post dialysis
Enalapril	5 - 40 mg qd	5 - 40 mg qd	2.5 - 40 mg qd	2.5 - 40 mg qd	2.5 - 10 mg
Fosinopril	10 - 40 mg qd	10 - 40 mg qd	10 - 40 mg qd	10 - 30 mg qd	none
Lisinopril	10 - 40 mg qd	10 - 40 mg qd	5 - 40 mg qd	2.5 - 40 mg qd	2.5 - 10 mg post dialysis
Perindopril	2 - 8 mg qd	2 - 8 mg qd	initial dose 2 mg	2 mg on dialysis days only	2 mg post dialysis
Quinapril	10 - 20 mg qd	10 - 20 mg qd	2.5 - 5 mg qd	2.5 - 5 mg qd	2.5 mg post dialysis
Ramipril	2.5 - 20 mg qd	2.5 - 20 mg qd	1.25 - 5 mg qd	1.25 - 5 mg qd	1.25

3. Angiotensin II receptor antagonists (No renal adjustment necessary):

Drug	Dose	Drug	Dose	Drug	Dose
Candesartan	8-32 mg qd	Irbesartan	150 - 300 mg qd	Losartan	25 - 100 mg qd
Telmisartan	40-80 mg/d	Valsartan	80 - 320 mg qd)		

4. Beta and alpha/beta adrenergic blockers

Drug	Normal	GFR > 50	GFR 10-50	GFR<10	Hemodialysis dose
Acebutolol	200 -800 mg qd (or divide bid)	200 -800 mg qd (or divide bid)	200 -400 mg qd (or divide bid)	200 mg qd	none
Atenolol	50 - 100 mg qd	50 - 100 mg qd	50 mg q 24 - 48h	25 mg q24 - 96h	25 - 50 mg
Betaxolol	10 - 20 mg qd	10 - 20 mg qd	10 - 20 mg qd	5 - 10 mg qd	none
Bisoprolol	5 - 20 mg qd	5 - 20 mg qd	Start at 2.5 mg and titrate with caution		none
Carteolol	2.5 - 10 mg qd	2.5 - 10 mg qd	2.5 - 10 mg q 48h	2.5 - 10 mg q 72h	

No renal adjustment necessary: Carvedilol (3.125 – 25 mg bid), Esmolol (50 - 150 µg/kg/min infusion), Labetolol (200 - 600 mg po q12h), Metoprolol (50 - 100 mg po q12h), Penbutolol (10 - 40 mg qd), Pindolol (10 - 40 mg qd), Propranolol (20 - 160 mg q 12h), Timolol (10 - 20 mg q12h)

5. Central agents

Drug	Normal	GFR > 50	GFR 10-50	GFR<10	Hemodialysis dose
Clonidine/chlorthalidone	Clonidine 0.1 – 0.3 mg/ Chlorthalidone 15 mg bid	Clonidine 0.1 – 0.3 mg/ Chlorthalidone 15 mg bid	Clonidine 0.1 – 0.3 mg/ Chlorthalidone 15 mg qd (adjustment for diuretic)	Clonidine 0.1 – 0.3 mg/ Chlorthalidone 15 mg q48 (adjustment for diuretic)	Contraindicated for anuria. Use alternative agent.
Methyldopa	250 –500 mg q6 –12 h (250 bid if combined with a non-thiazide antihypertensive)	250 – 500 mg q8	250 – 500 mg q 8 – 12h	250 – 500 mg q 12 - 24 h	250 mg post dialysis

No renal adjustment necessary:

Drug	Dosing	Drug	Dosing	Drug	Dosing
Clonidine	0.1 – 0.3 mg bid (1.2 mg bid is rarely used, maximum dose)	Guanfacine			1 - 2 mg qhs
Clonidine TTS	TTS – 1, TTS – 2, TTS – 3. Programmed delivery of 0.1, 0.2, or 0.3 mg clonidine per day for one week. Apply 1 – 2 patches weekly; adjust dose to BP.				

6. Vasodilators

Drug	Normal	GFR > 50	GFR 10-50	GFR<10	Hemodialysis dose
Hydralazine	25 – 50 mg q8h	25 – 50 mg q8h	25 – 50 mg q8h	25 - 50 mg q8 - 16h	none

No renal adjustment necessary: Diazoxide 150 - 300 mg bolus, Minoxidil 5 - 30 mg q 12h, Nitroprusside 0.25 - 8 µg/kg/min infusion

18d: Dosing and Renal Failure Adjustments for Commonly Prescribed Drugs (Cont.)

7. Calcium Channel Blockers
No renal adjustments necessary:

Drug (dihydropyridine)	Dosing
Amlodipine	5 - 10 mg qd
Felodipine sustained release	2.5 - 10 mg qd
Isradipine	5 - 10 mg qd
Nicardipine	20 - 30 mg q 8h
Nifedipine	10 - 30 mg q 8h or 30 - 120 mg qd (sustained release)
Nimodipine	30 mg q 8h
Nisoldipine sustained release	20 - 60 mg qd

Drug (non-dihydropyridine)	Dosing
Diltiazem	30 mg q6h to 120 mg q6 - 8h
Diltiazem sustained release	90 - 180 mg q12 or 180 - 480 mg qd (depending on preparation)
Verapamil	80 - 120 mg q 8h
Verapamil sustained release	180 mg q 24 - 240 mg q 12h

Oral antiarrhythmic agents

Drug	Normal	GFR > 50	GFR 10-50	GFR<10	Hemodialysis dose
Disopyramide	100 - 200 mg q6h or 200 - 300 mg extended release q12	100 - 200 mg q8h	100 - 200 mg q12 - 24h	100 - 200 mg q24 -40h	None
Flecainide	50 - 200 mg q 12h	50 - 200 mg q 12h	50 mg q 12h, adjust by level	50 mg q 12h or 100 mg qd, adjust by level	None
Mexiletine	150 - 300 mg q6-12h	150 - 300 mg q6-12h	150 - 300 mg q6-12h	150 - 250 mg q6-12h	None
Procainamide	25 mg/kg extended release q12h	25 mg/kg extended release q12h	350 - 400 mg regular procainamide q6 - 12h	350 - 400 mg regular procainamide q8 - 24h	200 mg
Quinidine	200 - 400 mg q 4 - 6h	200 - 400 mg q 4 - 6h	200 - 400 mg q 4 - 6h	200 - 300 mg q 4 - 6h	200 mg
Sotalol	80 - 160 mg q12h	80 - 160 mg q12h	80 - 160 mg q24 - 48h	Individualize	80 mg
Tocainide	400 - 600 mg q8h	400 - 600 mg q8h	400 - 600 mg q8h	200 - 400 mg q 8h	200 mg

No renal adjustment necessary: Moricizine (200 - 300 mg q8h), Propafenone (150 - 300 mg q8h)
Oral anti-arrhythmic agents should be adjusted to drug level and effect and should be prescribed by physicians familiar with their use.

Non-sedating antihistamines

Drug	Normal	GFR > 50	GFR 10-50	GFR<10	Hemodialysis dose
Cetirizine	5 - 20 mg qd	5 - 10 mg qd	5 mg qd (GFR < 30)	5 mg qd	none
Fexofenadine	60 mg q 12h	60 mg q 12h	60 mg q 12 - 24h	60 mg qd	none
Loratadine	10 mg qd	10 mg qd	10 mg q 48h (GFR < 30)	10 mg q 48h	none

No renal adjustment necessary: Astemizole (10 mg qd)

Gastrointestinal agents

1. H-2 blockers

Drug	Normal	GFR > 50	GFR 10-50	GFR<10	Hemodialysis dose
Cimetidine	400 mg q 12h or 400 - 800 mg qhs	400 mg q12h or 400 - 800 mg qhs	300 mg q12h	200 mg hs to 300 mg q12	none
Famotidine	20 - 40 mg qhs	20 mg qhs	20 mg qhs	20 mg q 24 - 48h	none
Nizatidine	150 - 300 mg qhs	150 - 300 mg qhs	150 mg qhs (GFR >20) maintenance: q 48h	150 mg q 48h (GFR-20) maintenance: q 72h	none
Ranitidine	150 q 12h or 300 mg qhs	150 q 12h or 300 mg qhs	150 mg qhs	150 mg qhs	time doses for post-dialysis

2. Proton pump inhibitors

No renal adjustment necessary: Lansoprazole (15 - 30 mg qd), Omeprazole (20 - 40 mg qd), Pantoprazole 40 mg QD, Proprazole 20 mg QD

18d: Dosing and Renal Failure Adjustments for Commonly Prescribed Drugs (*Cont.*)

Oral Hypoglycemic agents

Drug	Normal	GFR > 50	GFR 10-50	GFR<10	Hemodialysis dose
Acarbose	25 - 100 mg tid at start of meal	Avoid if creatinine > 2	Avoid	Avoid	
Acetohexamide	250 - 1500 mg qd	Avoid	Avoid	Avoid	
Chlorpropamide	100 - 500 mg qd	100 - 250 mg qd	Avoid	Avoid	
Glimepiride	1-8 mg qd	1-8 mg qd	1 mg qd (GFR-22)	1 mg qd	
Glyburide	1.25 - 20 mg qd (or divide bid)	Unknown	Avoid	Avoid	
Metformin	500 - 1000 mg bid with meals	Avoid	Avoid	Avoid	
Miglitol	25 - 100 mg tid	Unknown	Unknown	Unknown	
Repaglinide	0.5 - 2 mg TID after meals	Unknown	Unknown	Unknown	

No renal adjustment necessary: Glipizide (5 - 20 mg qd before breakfast), Pioglitazone (15 - 30 mg qd), Rosiglitazone (4 - 8 mg qd)Tolazamide (100 - 250 mg qd before breakfast), Tolbutamide
1 - 2 g qd before breakfast), Troglitazone 200 - 600 mg qd.
Adjust dose based on serum glucose and q 3 month HbA1C levels. See *Management of Diabetes*

Anticonvulsant agents
See *Management of Status Epilepticus* for intravenous dosing

Drug	Normal	GFR > 50	GFR 10-50	GFR<10	Hemodialysis dose
Gabapentin	300 - 800 mg q8h. Start 300 mg day 1, bid day 2, tid day 3.	400 mg q8h (GFR < 60)	300 mg q12h (GFR 30 - 60) 300 mg qd (GFR 14 - 30)	300 mg q48h	200 - 300 mg post each 4 hours of dialysis
Primidone	250 - 500 mg q6 - 8h. Start at 100 mg qhs day 1-3, then increase over 9 days.	250 - 500 mg q8h	250 - 500 mg q8-12h	250 - 500 mg q12-24h	1/3 dose
Topiramate	200 - 800 mg q12h. Start at 50 mg qhs, increase over 8 weeks		50% of usual dose (GFR < 70)		Supplemental dose post dialysis

No renal adjustments necessary:

Drug	Dosing
Carbamazepine	200 mg q12h to 400 tid or 600 mg q12 (XR)
Ethosuximide	500 - 1500 mg qd
Felbamate	400 - 1200 mg tid

Drug	Dosing
Phenytoin	1000 mg load, then 200 - 400 mg qd
Valproic acid	15 - 60 mg/kg/d. If >250 mg, divide bid

Bennett WM et al. Drug Prescribing in Renal Failure: Dosing guidelines for adults, 3rd ed. American College of Physicians, Philadelphia, 1994
Physicians Desk Reference. Medical Economics Co., Montvale NJ, 2000, www.pdr.net,
Micromedex.

Index